1 Introduction

S hamanism is the oldest religion on the planet!

In human existence it predates current day organized religions by many millennia. Shamans are traditional healers, guides and protectors. They are a universal expression of the interaction between people and the natural and supernatural worlds. European cave paintings and carvings showing shaman date from the Paleolithic era and in 2016, a12,000-year-old grave of a female shaman has been uncovered in Israel.

Shamans have played an essential role in the defence of the psychic integrity of their community for thousands of years. They defend life, health, fertility, and the world of "light," against death, diseases, sterility, disaster and the world of "darkness." Fundamental is the shaman's struggle against what we could call the powers of evil. Shamans cannot foresee the future, but change the outcome. As an example, shamans can find out where food or game is located, or averting threats. This is a vital difference between shamanism and clairvoyance.[1]

These skills and abilities helped and protected their communities. However, when their dances, songs, and ceremonies were witnessed by ill-informed missionaries of western Abrahamic religions they were labelled as being possessed by the devil when those applying the label had no comprehension, or, understanding of what an Altered State of Consciousness is.

In this book we look at what a Pagan and Paganism is and why some historic cultures such as Roman or Greek have "mythologies" when in fact they were pagan animistic and polytheistic cultures but rarely called out for it today.

We look at what a shaman and shamanism are and how they have developed through different ages of absorption and persecution.

Connect with our Private Facebook group to learn more about Reiki. Click here.

Subscribe to our newsletter to learn more about Reiki and Shamanism. Click here

Enjoy.

Mark Ashford, MSc,
Usui Tibetan Reiki Master and Teacher [IARP], Registered Reiki Teacher and Practitioner [CRA]
https://www.markaashford.com

---

[1] https://www.energy-shifter.com/shamanism-and-spiritual-techniques.html, Shamanism,andsoulretrieval-SpiritualHouseCleansing.

2   Table of Contents

3 Table of Figures

4   Paganism and Related Beliefs

Before we look at Shamans and Paganism, we need to understand what Paganism is, not what it is represented as today, or through the eyes of organized Abrahamic religions.

Paganism is a term first used in the fourth century by early Christians for people in the Roman Empire who practised polytheism. This was because they were increasingly rural relative to the Christian population, or because they were not milites Christi—soldiers of Christ. Alternate terms in Christian texts for the same group were Hellenes, gentile, and heathen. Ritual sacrifice was an integral part of ancient Greco-Roman religion and was regarded as a sign of whether a person was pagan or Christian.[2]

Paganism was originally a pejorative and derogatory term for polytheism, implying its inferiority. Paganism has broadly connoted as the "religion of the peasantry." During and after the Middle Ages, the term paganism applied to any unfamiliar religion, and the term presumed a belief in false God or Gods. Most modern pagan religions exist today. Modern or Neopaganism expresses a world view that is pantheistic, polytheistic or animistic; some are monotheistic. [3]

4.1   Paganism

The term paganism covers a great number of spiritual and religious beliefs, a follower or practitioner of those beliefs can cause them being referred to as pagan. Pagan is a term often used by adherents of Abrahamic[4] religions, especially Catholic missionaries who denigrated and continue to malign and persecute local traditional religions and healing practices.

The Abrahamic religions, also referred to collectively as Abrahamism, is a group of Semitic-originated religious communities of faith that claim descent from the Judaism of the ancient Israelites and the worship of the God of Abraham. The Abrahamic religions are monotheistic, with the term deriving from the patriarch Abraham a major biblical figure from the Old Testament, who is recognized by Jews, Christians, Muslims, and others.[5]

Another definition of Abrahamic religion is a term used to group Christianity and Judaism together, either regarding Christianity's derivation from Judaism, both religions' common use of the Bible, or because of perceived parallels or commonalities and shared values between the two religions.[6] Another variation on these definitions is any religious act, practice, or ceremony which is not Christian. Jews and Muslims use the term to refer to anyone outside *their* religion.

Still others Paganism as being a religion outside of Christianity, Judaism, Hinduism, and Buddhism, while some simply define it as being without an organized Abrahamic religion.

The word pagan is derived from the Latin word, paganus, which means a country dweller.[7]

---

[2] Wikipedia, Paganism.
[3] Wikipedia, Paganism.
[4] Wikipedia, Abrahamicreligions.
[5] Wikipedia, Abrahamicreligions.
[6] Wikipedia, Judeo-Christian.
[7] https://www.allaboutspirituality.org/paganism.htm, Paganism.

As Christianity progressed into the present age, a pagan became anyone not being a Christian, and paganism denoted a non-Christian belief or religion. If the religion did not fit into the Judeo-Christian-Islamic or Eastern mould, then one practising that religion was said to be involved in paganism. [8]

Certainly, when Orthodox Christians spread into Siberia, Mongolia and Tibet, they persecuted "pagan" practitioners, especially local community shaman healers.

The primary marker of Paganism is the belief in over one God!

Some of those in ancient times, who are called Pagans today, believed there was not just one god but several gods and goddesses. The stories from Greek mythology are famous examples of pagan religion. Add to the Greek Stories those of the Romans, the Mongols, The Vikings, Egyptians and the Incas to name a few.

Pagans usually focus on spirituality and nature, rather than on doctrines and dogma. Not all pagans are polytheists, they believe in over one God. Some of them are monotheists. They believe in only one god. Though the god is not Judeo-Christian.

The term heathen is derived from Old English. It is an Anglo-Saxon word from the fifth century AD. It was used to refer to someone who is non-Christian or Jewish, the only organized religions in England.

Pagans may be trained in particular traditions or they may follow their own inspiration. Paganism is not dogmatic. Pagans pursue their own vision of the divine as a direct and personal experience.

The term has recently been revived in the forms Heathenry and Heathenism, often but not always capitalized, as alternative names for the Germanic neopagan[9] movement, adherents of which may self-identify as heathens. Neo-druids would fit into the neo-pagan category and can be seen celebrating at Stonehenge at the various times of the year. Neo-Druidism includes the Ancient Order of druids, and, the druid Order.

Interestingly enough, Hinduism[10], a religion of the Indian subcontinent with approximately 1.25 billion followers or 15–16% of the global population has over 30 million gods and goddesses and is not considering Pagan.

Some keynotes for understanding Paganism:

Comparison with Abrahamic Religions

Abrahamic Religion	Paganism
Professes one God	Professes many gods or none
A centralized text that contains God's words or messages	No central text or set of beliefs

---

[8] https://www.allaboutspirituality.org/paganism.htm, Paganism.
[9] Wikipedia, ListofNeopaganmovements.
[10] Wikipedia, Hinduism.

Abrahamic Religion	Paganism
Jesus, as God's son, came to earth as a baby and died on the cross for the global sins of humankind and rose again.	Some pagan beliefs include Jesus but do not put the emphasis on him as Abrahamic Religions do

4.2   Characteristics of Paganism

The following characteristics are taken from The Pagan Federation International website—https://www.paganfederation.org/what-is-paganism/ and Wikipedia as noted in the footnotes

- Nature—Veneration[11]

  The spirit of place is recognized in Pagan religion, whether as a personified natural feature such as a mountain, lake or spring, or as a fully articulated guardian divinity such as, for example, Athena, the goddess of Athens.

  The cycle of the natural year, with the different emphasis brought by its different seasons, is seen by most Pagans as a model of spiritual growth and renewal, and as a sequence marked by festivals [summer and winter solstice] which offer access to different divinities according to their affinity with different times of year.

  Many Pagans see the Earth itself as sacred: in ancient Greece the Earth was always offered the first libation of wine, although she had no priesthood and no temple.

- Polytheism: Pluralism and Diversity[12]

  Polytheism is the worship of or belief in multiple deities, which are usually assembled into a pantheon of gods and goddesses, along with their own religions and rituals. In most religions which accept polytheism, the different gods and goddesses are representations of forces of nature or ancestral principles, and can be viewed either as autonomous or as aspects or emanations of a creator deity or transcendental absolute principle monistic theologies, which manifests immanently in nature pantheistic and pantheistic theologies. Most of the polytheistic deities of ancient religions, with the notable exceptions of the Ancient Egyptian and Hindu deities, were conceived as having physical bodies.[13]

  The many deities of Paganism are a recognition of the diversity of Nature. Some Pagans see the goddesses and gods as a community of individuals, much like the diverse human community in this world. Others, such as followers of Isis and Osiris from ancient times onwards, and Wiccan-based Pagans in the modern world, see all the goddesses as one Great Goddess, and all the gods as one Great God, whose harmonious interaction is the secret of the universe. Yet others think there is a supreme divine principle, that "both want and do not want to be called Zeus," as Heraclitus wrote in the fifth century BC. Or which the Great Goddess Mother of All Things, as Isis, was to the first century CE novelist Apuleius and the Great Goddess is to many Western Pagans nowadays. Yet others, such as the Emperor Julian, the great restorer of Paganism in Christian antiquity, and many

---

[11] Pagan Federation International, WhatisPaganism.
[12] International, WhatisPaganism.
[13] Wikipedia, Polytheism.

Hindu mystics nowadays, believe in an abstract Supreme Principle, the origin and source of all things.

But even these last Pagans recognize that other spiritual beings, although perhaps one with a greater being, are themselves divine, and are not false or partial divinities. Pagans who worship the one are described as henotheists, believers in a supreme divine principle, rather than monotheists, believers in one true deity beside which all other deities are false.

- The Goddess[14]

Pagan religions all recognize the feminine face of divinity. A religion without goddesses can hardly be classified as Pagan. Some pagan paths, such as the cult of Odin or of Mithras, offer exclusive allegiance to one male god. But they do not deny the reality of other gods and goddesses, as monotheists do. (The word "cult" has always meant the specialized veneration of one particular deity or pantheon, and has only recently been extended to mean the worship of a deified or semi-divine human leader.) Non-pagan religions, such as Judaism, Christianity and Islam, often but not always, abhor the very idea of female divinity. The (then) Anglican Bishop of London even said a few years ago that religions with goddesses were "degenerate"!

- The Horned God[15]

The Horned god is one of the two primary deities found in Wicca and some related forms of Neopaganism. The term horned god itself predates Wicca, and is an early 20th-century syncretic term for a horned or antlered anthropomorphic god partly based on historical horned deities.

The Horned god represents the male part of the religion's duotheistic theological system, the consort of the female triple goddess of the Moon or other Mother goddess. In common Wiccan belief, he is associated with nature, wilderness, sexuality, hunting, and the life cycle. Whilst depictions of the deity vary, he is always shown with either horns or antlers upon his head, often depicted as being thermophilic (having a beast's head), in this way emphasizing "the union of the divine and the animal," the latter of which includes humanity.

In traditional Wicca—British Traditional Wicca, he is regarded as a dualistic god of twofold aspects: bright and dark, night and day, summer and winter, the Oak King and the Holy King. In this dualistic view, his two horns symbolize, in part, his dual nature. Using horns to symbolize duality is also reflected in the phrase, "on the horns of a dilemma." The three aspects of the Goddess and the two aspects of the Horned god are sometimes mapped on to the five points of the pentagram, although which points correspond to which deity aspects vary. In some other systems, he is represented as a triune god, split into three aspects that reflect those of the Triple goddess: The Youth (Warrior), the Father, and the Sage.

- Other Characteristics[16]

---

[14] International, WhatisPaganism.
[15] Wikipedia, HornedGod.
[16] Wikipedia, HornedGod.

The many divinities of pagan religion often include ancestral deities. The Anglo-Saxon royal houses of England traced their ancestry back to a god, usually Woden, and the Celtic kings of Cumbria traced their descent from the god Beli and the goddess Anna. Local and national heroes and heroines may be deified, as was Julius Caesar, and in all pagan societies, the deities of the household are venerated. These may include revered ancestors and, for a while, the newly dead, who may or may not choose to leave the world of the living for good. They may include local spirits of place, either as personified individuals such as the spirit of a spring or the house's guardian toad or snake, or as group spirits such as Elves in England, the Little People in Ireland, Kobolds in Germany, Barstuccae in Lithuania, Lares and Penates in ancient Rome, and so on. A household shrine focuses on the cult of these deities, and there is usually an annual ritual to honour them. The spirit of the hearth is often venerated, sometimes with a daily offering of food and drink, sometimes with an annual ritual of extinguishing and relighting the fire. Through ancestral and domestic ritual, a spirit of continuity is preserved, and by the transmission of characteristics and purposes from the past, the future is assured of meaning.

So, not all pagan religion is public religion; much is domestic. And not all pagan deities are humanoid super-people; many are elemental or collective. We are looking at a religion which pervades the whole of everyday life.

One consequence of the veneration of Nature, the outlook which sees Nature as a manifestation of divinity rather than as a neutral or inanimate object, is that divination and magic are accepted parts of life. Augury, divination by interpreting the flight of birds, was widespread in the ancient world and is in modern pagan societies, as is extispicy, divination by reading the entrails of the sacrificed animal, itself a larger scale version of divination by reading the tea-leaves left in a teacup. As well as reading the signs already given by deities, diviners may also actively ask the universe to send a sign, e.g., by casting stones to read the geomantic patterns into which they fall, by casting runes or the yarrow stalks of the I Ching. Pagans usually believe that the divine world will answer a genuine request for information. Trance seership and mediumship are also used to communicate with the Otherworld.

Magic, the deliberate production of results in this world by Otherworld means, is accepted as a workable activity in pagan societies, since the two worlds are thought to be in constant communication. In ancient Rome, a new bride would ceremonially anoint the doorposts of her new home with a wolf's fat to keep famine from the household, and her newborn child would be given a consecrated amulet to wear as a protection against harmful spirits. The Norse warriors of the Viking age would cast the magical "war fetter" upon their enemies to paralyze them, and Anglo-Saxon manuscripts record spells to bring healing and fertility. Specialist magical technologists such as horse whisperers and healers are common throughout pagan societies, but often the practice of magic for unfair personal gain or for harm to another is forbidden, exactly as physical extortion and assault are forbidden everywhere.

- Modern Paganism[17]

---

[17] Wikipedia, HornedGod.

With its respect for plurality, the refusal to judge other ways of life as wrong simply because they differ from one's own, with its veneration of a natural (and supernatural) world from which Westerners in the age of technology have become increasingly isolated, and with its respect for women and the feminine principle as embodied in the many goddesses of the various pantheons, Paganism has much to offer people of European background today. Hence, it is being taken up by them in large numbers. When they realize it is, in fact, their ancestral heritage, its attraction grows.

Democracy, for example, was pioneered by the ancient Athenians and much later reinvented by the Pagan colonizers of Iceland, home of Europe's oldest parliament. Our modern love of the arts was fostered in Pagan antiquity, with its pageants and its temples, but had no place in iconoclastic Christianity and Islam. The development of science as we know it began in the desire of the Greeks and Babylonians to understand the hidden patterns of Nature, and the cultivation of humane urbanity, the ideal of the well-rounded, cultured personality, was imported by Renaissance thinkers from the writings of Cicero. In the Pagan cities of the Mediterranean lands, the countryside was never far from people's awareness, with parks, gardens and even zoos, all reintroduced into modern Europe, not by the religions of the book, and not by utilitarian atheists, but by the classically inspired planners of the Enlightenment.

In the present day, the Pagan tradition manifests both as communities reclaiming their ancient sites and ceremonies (especially in Eastern Europe), to put humankind back in harmony with the Earth, and as individuals pursuing a personal spiritual path alone or in a small group (especially in Western Europe and the European-settled countries abroad), under the tutelage of one of the Pagan divinities. To most modern Pagans in the West, the whole of life is to be affirmed joyfully and without shame, as long as other people are not harmed by one's own tastes. Modern Pagans are relaxed and at ease with themselves and others, and women have a dignity which is not always found outside pagan circles.

Modern Pagans, not tied down either by the customs of an established religion or by the dogmas of a revealed one, are often creative, playful and individualistic, affirming the importance of the individual psyche as it interfaces with a greater power. There is a respect for all of life and usually a desire to participate with rather than to dominate other beings. What playwright Eugene O'Neil called "the creative pagan acceptance of life" is at the forefront of the modern movement. This is bringing something new to religious life and to social behaviour, a way of pluralism without fragmentation, of creativity without anarchy, of wisdom without dogma. Here is an age-old current surfacing in a new form suited to the needs of the present day.

4.3 Pagan Traditions [18]

Wicca Traditions
British Traditional Wicca
Gardnerian Wicca (1954)
Alexandrian Wicca (1967)
Central Valley Wicca (1969)
Algard Wicca (1972)
Chthonioi Alexandrian Wicca (1974)
Blue Star Wicca (1975)
Eclectic Wicca and Inclusive Wicca
Celtic Wicca
Saxon Wicca
Dianic Wicca
McFarland Dianic Wicca
Faery Wicca
Georgian Wicca
Ulyssean Wicca
Wiccan church
New Reformed Orthodox Order of the Golden Dawn (1968)
Church and School of Wicca (1968)
Circle Sanctuary (1974)
Covenant of the Goddess (1975)
Aquarian Tabernacle Church (1979)
Rowan Tree Church (1979)
Covenant of Unitarian Universalist Pagans (1985)
Coven of the Far-Flung Net (1998)

---

[18] Wikipedia, ListofNeopaganmovements.

New Age, eclectic or syncretic
Church of All Worlds
Church of Aphrodite
Christian Wicca
Feraferia
Goddess movement
Huna
Neoshamanism
Pagan Federation
Radical Faeries
Universal Pantheist Society

Other Pagan Traditions
Stregheria (Italian tradition)
Hedge Witchcraft
Cochrane's Craft
Children of Artemis
Feri Tradition
Reclaiming

Figure 1. Vikings on their Longboat

5   Vikings

The Vikings originated from what today are the Scandinavian countries of Denmark, Norway, and Sweden.

In the history of Europe, the Middle Ages or Medieval Period lasted from the 5th to the 15th century. During the Middle Ages, we have many other "ages" or periods. Notable is the Viking Age[19] which lasted from AD 800 to AD 1050.

The Viking age was characterized by a people who were technologically, militarily and culturally advanced by the time the Viking Age dawned. These advantages allowed the Vikings to travel far. By sailing their flat-bottomed ships down the Danube, they reached the Black Sea, between Eastern Europe, the Caucasus, and Western Asia. The y visited the Mediterranean and North Afrika.

Several factors, not one reason, drove them to undertake these voyages of discovery and raiding.

The landscape of Scandinavia, especially Norway, is rough. The fjords provide little farming land or riches and to get to a community only a short distance away as the crow flies is tortuous and difficult to travel across the rocky and mountainous dividing land. Far easier to sail around the end of the fjord into the next one. They had the boats and the sailing experience and expertise to make open sea voyages possible.

Another factor that has been put forward was the polygynous nature of Viking society. If you were a rich and powerful chieftain, you would have multiple wives and concubines. The low number of women for men who were not so wealthy or powerful led to them undertaking voyages and raids could provide wealth, or women, or both.

In Denmark and Sweden, which did not have such a hostile landscape as Norway, migrating tribes and peoples were invading and taking land from them. This put pressure on the existing tribes that to find another location in which to grow and thrive.

Another explanation is that the Vikings exploited a moment of weakness in the surrounding regions. England suffered from internal divisions and was relatively easy prey given the proximity of many towns to the sea or to navigable rivers. Lack of organized naval opposition throughout Western Europe allowed Viking ships to travel freely, raiding or trading as opportunity permitted. The decline in the profitability of old trade routes could also have played a role. Trade between western Europe and the rest of Eurasia suffered a severe blow when the Western Roman Empire fell in the 5th century. The expansion of Islam in the seventh century had also affected trade with western Europe.[20]

The Vikings raids on England were not the first, three centuries before the Vikings, the Jutes invaded England and the British Isles. The Saxons and the Angles did the same, embarking from mainland Europe. The Viking raids were, however, the first to be documented in writing by eyewitnesses, and they were much larger in scale and frequency than in previous times.[21]

_____

[19] Wikipedia, VikingAge.
[20] Wikipedia, Vikings.
[21] Wikipedia, Vikings.

Viking Mythology or Viking Paganism includes a pantheon of several hundred Gods, Goddesses, Giants, elves and other creatures. The most powerful and well known are.

5.1 Odin

One eyed the most powerful of the Viking Gods. Associated with war and death, he is also the most intelligent. While he has one eye, the eye that remains is as bright as the sun. The eye that is missing was sacrificed so that he could drink from the fountain of wisdom.

Odin is the father of several other Viking Gods such as Thor and Loki.

5.2 Thor

He is the God of Thunder; he has a long-bearded and red hair. During thunderstorms, Vikings believed it was Thor riding through the heavens on his chariot and it was his hammer that making the thunderstorm noises.

He is renowned for protecting both the Gods and Humans from various forms of evil.

In Norse mythology, when the last battle between good and evil is fought on the day of Ragnarok, Thor will slay the Midgard serpent but will also die from the serpent's poison.

In the days of the week, Thursday is named after Thor, or Thorsday.

5.3 Loki

Both clever and malicious, he is brother to Thor, but does all he can to cause the fall of the Norse Gods. He is the most powerful magician in Norse mythology and it is using this magic that he forces Norse gods to suffer many losses.

He causes the death of Balder, one of the most popular of Norse gods, and then refuses to repent for his actions. This leads to the Norse doomsday, whereby Norse Gods are pitted against the forces of evil in a last battle. Loki dies, fighting against the gods, as do several notable Norse gods.

5.4 Freya

Her husband or mate is Odin. Because of the polygamous nature of the Viking world, she is not the mother of Thor and Loki, Odin's other wives, Frigg is their mother.

Freya is famous for her fondness of love, fertility, beauty, and fine material possessions—and, because of these predilections, she's considered being the "party girl" of the Viking Aesir gods.

Freya is the archetype of the völva, a professional or semi-professional practitioner of seidr[22], the most organized form of Norse magic. It was she who first brought this art to the gods, and, by extension, to humans as well. Given her expertise in controlling and manipulating the desires,

---

[22] Wikipedia, Seidr.

health, and prosperity of others, she is a being whose knowledge, and power are almost without equal.

Freya is also reputed to travel Viking battle fields in a chariot pulled by two large cats. She is searching for worthy and valiant souls of fallen Vikings whom she takes back to eternal merriment in Valhalla.

Seidr is pre-Christian Norse magic and shamanism that involved discerning the course of fate and working within its structure to bring about change, often by symbolically weaving new events into being. This power might be put to any use imaginable, and examples cover virtually the entire range of the human condition can be found in Old Norse literature.

In the days of the week, Friday is named after Freya, or Freya's Day.

6 Roman Paganism

Ancient Romans honoured a wide variety of gods, and many are still worshiped today by Roman reconstruction groups. To the Romans, their deities were a part of daily life, and influenced it accordingly. The Gods and Goddesses were not merely to be worshiped in times of need.

For example, if someone were undertaking a journey, an offering or prayer would be devoted to the Goddess of travel; Abeona protected travellers from the outward part of their journey. The Goddess Adiona protected travellers on their homeward journey. In addition, Mercury was a Roman god who aided travellers.

Besides these Gods and Goddesses, smaller, less well-known local gods and goddesses were also venerated. For example, a shrine might have been set up at a river crossing after it was determined a certain God or Goddess ruled over the crossing. A traveller would make an offering and payer at the shrine for a safe river crossing.

Many modern Pagans observe festivals and celebrations that originated in the classical Roman calendar.

Early Roman Paganism was tied closely to daily life, and it wasn't uncommon for people to celebrate different gods and goddesses every month or even weekly. Even if your path isn't specifically rooted in Roman religion, you can still observe these holidays, many of which were based on seasonal or agricultural markers.

Here are some of the best-known gods and goddesses of the ancient Romans:

6.1 Bacchus

Dionysus[23] or Dionysos is the god of the grape harvest, winemaking and wine, of fertility, orchards and fruit, vegetation, insanity, ritual madness, religious ecstasy, festivity and theatre in ancient Greek religion and myth.

He is also known as Bacchus the name adopted by the Romans; the frenzy he induces is bakkheia. His thyrsus, sometimes wounds with ivy and dripping with honey, is both a beneficent wand and a weapon used to destroy those who oppose his cult and the freedoms he represents. As Eleutherios ("the liberator"), his wine, music and ecstatic dance to free his followers from self-conscious fear and care, and subvert the oppressive restraints of the powerful. Those who partake of his mysteries are believed to become possessed and empowered by the god himself. [24]

6.2 Cybele

An Anatolian mother Goddess. Rome adopted and developed a particular form of her cult after the Sibylline oracle in 205 BC recommended her conscription as a key religious ally in Rome's second war against Carthage (218 to 201 BC). [25]

---

[23] Wikipedia, Dionysus.
[24] Wikipedia, Dionysus.
[25] Wikipedia, Cybele.

Roman mythographers reinvented her as a Trojan goddess, and thus an ancestral goddess of the Roman people by the Trojan prince Aeneas. As Rome eventually established hegemony over the Mediterranean world, Romanized forms of Cybele's cults spread throughout Rome's empire. Greek and Roman writers debated and disputed the meaning and morality of her cults and priesthoods, which remain controversial subjects in modern scholarship. [26]

6.3 Janus

In ancient Roman religion and myth, Janus is the god of beginnings, gates, transitions, time, duality, doorways, passages, and endings. He is usually depicted as having two faces, since he looks to the future and to the past. The month of January is named for Janus but according to ancient Roman farmers' almanacs Juno was the tutelary deity of the month.[27]

Janus presided over the beginning and ending of conflict, and hence war and peace. The gates of a building in Rome named after him (not a temple, as it is often called, but an open enclosure with gates at each end) were opened in time of war, and closed to mark peace (which did not happen very often). As a god of transitions, he had functions pertaining to birth journeys and exchange, and in his association with Portunus, a similar harbour and gateway God, he was concerned with travelling, trading and shipping. [28]

6.4 Mars

In ancient Roman religion and myth, Mars was the god of war and also an agricultural guardian, a combination characteristic of early Rome.[29] He was also the father with Rhea Silvia of Romulus and Remus, the mythical founders of Rome.

In today's calendar, March is named after him and many festivals were conducted in his honour in that month. Festivals also took place in October, which was the start of the military campaigning season in Rome. He represented military power to secure peace and was a father of the Roman people.

Of course, as God of War, the planet Mars is named after him.

---

[26] Wikipedia, Cybele.
[27] Wikipedia, Janus.
[28] Wikipedia, Janus.
[29] Wikipedia, Mars.

7 Greek Paganism

Ancient Greek religion includes a collection of beliefs, rituals, and mythology originating in ancient Greece as both popular public religion and cult practices. These groups varied enough for it to be possible to speak of Greek religions or "cults" in the plural, though most of them shared similarities.[30]

Most ancient Greeks recognized the twelve major Olympian gods and goddesses—Zeus, Hera, Poseidon, Demeter, Athena, Ares, Aphrodite, Apollo, Artemis, Hephaestus, Hermes, and either Hestia or Dionysus—although philosophies such as Stoicism and some forms of Platonism used language that seems to assume a single transcendent deity. The worship of these deities, and several others, were found across the Greek world, though they often have different epithets that distinguished aspects of the deity, and often reflect the absorption of other local deities into the Panhellenic scheme. [31]

Partly because of geographic closeness and the influence of Ancient Greek Religion over religions in the Mediterranean, Greek influence on Rome and the evolution of Roman Pagan Gods and Goddesses was significant.

Here are some of the best-known gods and goddesses of the ancient Greeks:

7.1 Aphrodite

The goddess of love and romance.

She was honoured by the ancient Greeks and is still celebrated by many modern Pagans. According to legend, she was born fully formed from the white sea form that arose when the god Uranus was castrated. She came ashore on the island of Cyprus, and later was married off by Zeus to Hephaistos, the deformed artisan of Olympus. A festival was held regularly to honour Aphrodite, appropriately called the aphrodisiac. An aphrodisiac to this day is referred to as a food, drug, potion, or other agents that arouses sexual desire.[32]

7.2 Ares

Son of Zeus and Hera, Ares was the god of war. Renowned for his own exploits and adventures in battle, he was also an agent of justice when he became embroiled in disputes with other Gods.

7.3 Artemis

A huntress, Artemis, like her twin brother Apollo, possessed a wide variety of attributes. She is still honoured by some pagan followers as an agent of change and female transition. Artemis was also the Greek goddess of childbirth, protecting women in labour, but she could also bring them sickness and death. Many cults dedicated to Artemis appeared around the ancient Greek world. Most were connected to childbirth, puberty, and motherhood.

---

[30] Wikipedia, AncientGreekreligion.
[31] Wikipedia, AncientGreekreligion.
[32] Dictionary.com, Aphrodisiac.

7.4   Athena

Goddess of war appears I Greek legend as a helper of various heroes and in their legends. Heroes, such as Heracles, Odysseus and Jason, all received help from Athena.

Although identified as a warrior goddess, she did not fill the same role as Ares, who approached war muscularly and in a frenzy of action and battle. Instead, Athena helped warriors make considered and wise choices that will eventually lead to victory.

Athena did not have lovers and was often revered as a virgin goddess/warrior.

7.5   Eros

The god of lust and pleasure; the word erotic is rooted in his name, and his primal sexual hunger and desire. Mythology describes him as the son of Aphrodite and Ares. Eros and Aphrodite are often worshiped together.

7.6   Gaia

Life force is the root energy from which all beings arise. These include the earth, sea, and mountains. Gaia is a female energy that energy is concentrated in some locations that are sacred even today. Many Pagans and Wiccans honour Gaia today.

7.7   Zeus

Like Odin, Zeus was the preeminent ruler of all Greek Gods. He is a provider of justice and law from Mount Olympus, where the Greek Gods live. Married to Hera, he is known for his laciferous ways. Greek or Hellenic Pagans still worship and honour him.

According to the traditional understanding, Kabbalah dates from Eden. It came down from a remote past as a revelation to elect Tzadikim—righteous people, and, mostly, was preserved only by a privileged few. Talmudic Judaism records its view of the proper protocol for teaching this wisdom, as well as many of its concepts, in the Talmud, Tractate Hagigah, 11b-13a, "One should not teach … the Act of Creation in pairs, nor the Act of the Chariot to an individual, unless he is wise and can understand the implications himself, etc."[33]

Kabbalah is an esoteric method, discipline, and school of thought in Jewish mysticism. A traditional Kabbalist in Judaism is called a Mequbbāl. The definition of Kabbalah varies according to the tradition and aims of those following it, from its religious origin as an integral part of Judaism, to its later adaptations in Western esotericism—Christian Kabbalah and Hermetic Qabalah. The esoteric teachings explain the relationship between the unchanging god—the mysterious Ein Sof[34], "The Infinite" and the mortal, finite universe God's creation. It forms the foundation of mystical religious interpretations within Judaism.

Jewish Kabbalists originally developed their own transmission of sacred texts within the realm of Jewish tradition, and often use classical Jewish scriptures to explain and show its mystical teachings. These teachings are held by followers in Judaism to define the inner meaning of both the Hebrew Bible and traditional rabbinic literature and their formerly concealed transmitted dimension, as well as to explain the significance of Jewish religious observances. One of the fundamental kabbalistic texts, the Zohar, was first published in the 13th century, and the almost universal form adhered to in modern Judaism is Lurianic Kabbalah.[35]

Traditional practitioners believe its earliest origins predate world religions, forming the primordial blueprint for Creation's philosophies, religions, sciences, arts, and political systems.

Historically, Kabbalah emerged after earlier forms of Jewish mysticism, in 12th- to 13th-century Spain and Southern France, and was reinterpreted during the Jewish mystical renaissance of 16th-century Ottoman Palestine. [36]

Isaac Luria is considered the father of contemporary Kabbalah; Lurianic Kabbalah was popularized as Hasidic Judaism from the 18th century onwards. [3] During the 20th century, academic interest in kabbalistic texts led primarily by the Jewish historian Gershom Scholem has inspired the development of historical research on Kabbalah in Judaic studies.[37]

---

[33] Wikipedia, Kabbalah.
[34] Wikipedia, EinSof.
[35] Wikipedia, Kabbalah.
[36] Wikipedia, Kabbalah.
[37] Wikipedia, Kabbalah.

9 Egyptian Paganism

Egyptian or "Kemet" mythology, Kemet being the ancient name for Egypt includes many Gods and goddesses. Some are beings who are part human, part animal. There are over 2,000 deities in the Egyptian or Kemetic pantheon. In the same way as the Greeks and Romans included worship and honouring of the deities in everyday life, so did the Ancient Egyptians.

Egyptian Ethics is based on ancient Egyptian texts. The most commonly referred to being the Declaration of Innocence, also called the "Negative Confessions." This contains forty-two sins a deceased person claims not to have done. The other most commonly referred to text is the Wisdom Texts, which are pieces of advice written by Ancient Egyptians.

To do good is doing Ma'at, or what is right, just, and orderly.

9.1   Osiris

King of Egyptian Gods

Osiris is the god of a wide range of attributes, fertility, agriculture, the afterlife, the dead, resurrection, life, and vegetation in ancient Egyptian religion.[38]

Classically depicted as a green-skinned deity with a pharaoh's beard, partially mummy-wrapped at the legs, wearing a distinctive Atef[39] crown, and holding a symbolic crook and flail[40] traditional symbols of pharaonic authority.

He was one of the first to be associated with the mummy wrap. When his brother, Set, cut him up into pieces after killing him, Isis, his wife, found all the pieces and wrapped his body. Osiris was considered the eldest son of the god Geb and the sky goddess Nut, as well as being the brother and husband of Isis, with Horus being considered his posthumously begotten son. [41]

He was also associated with the epithet Khenti-Amentiu, meaning "Foremost of the Westerners," a reference to his kingship in the land of the dead. Through syncretism with Iah, he is also a god of the Moon. [42]

He is known as the god who taught humanity the secrets of civilization. Today, he is honoured by some Pagans as a god of the underworld and of the harvest.

9.2   Isis

Isis was first mentioned in the Old Kingdom c. 2686–2181 BCE as one of the main characters of the Osiris myth, in which she resurrects her slain husband, the divine king Osiris, and produces and protects his heir, Horus. She was believed to help the dead enter the afterlife as she had

---

[38] Wikipedia, Osiris.
[39] Wikipedia, Atef.
[40] Wikipedia, Crookandflail.
[41] Wikipedia, Osiris.
[42] Wikipedia, Osiris.

helped Osiris, and she was considered the divine mother of the pharaoh, who was likened to Horus.[43]

Her maternal aid was invoked in healing spells to benefit ordinary people. Originally, she played a limited role in royal rituals and temple rites, although she was more prominent in funerary practices and magical texts.[44]

She was usually portrayed in art as a human woman wearing a throne-like hieroglyph on her head. During the New Kingdom (c. 1550–1070 BCE), as she took on traits that originally belonged to Hathor, the preeminent goddess of earlier times, Isis was portrayed wearing Hathor's headdress: a sun disc between the horns of a cow.

In the first millennium BCE, Osiris and Isis became the most widely worshiped Egyptian deities, and Isis absorbed traits from many other goddesses. Rulers in Egypt and its neighbour to the south, Nubia, built temples dedicated primarily to Isis, and her temple at Philae was a religious centre for Egyptians and Nubians alike.

Her reputed magical power was greater than that of all other gods, and she was said to protect the kingdom from its enemies, govern the skies and the natural world, and have power over fate itself. She was the divine mother of every pharaoh of Egypt, and ultimately of Egypt itself.

9.3   Hathor

Patron of Women

In Egyptian religion, Hathor was a predynastic goddess who embodied femininity, love, and the joy of motherhood. Besides being a symbol of fertility, she was known as a goddess of the underworld, in that she welcomed the newly departed to the West.

9.4   Horus

9.5   The Falcon Headed God

Horus, the falcon-headed god, is a familiar ancient Egyptian god. He has become one of the most commonly used symbols of Egypt, seen on Egyptian airplanes, and on hotels and restaurants throughout the land.

Horus is the son of Osiris and Isis, the divine child of the Holy Family triad. He is one of many gods associated with the falcon. His name means "he who is above" and "he who is distant." The falcon had been worshiped from the earliest times as a cosmic deity whose body represents the heavens and whose eyes represent the sun and the moon. Horus is depicted as a falcon wearing a crown with a cobra or the Double Crown of Egypt. The hooded cobra (uraeus), which the gods and pharaohs wore on their foreheads, symbolizes light and royalty. It is there to protect the person from harm.

---

[43] Wikipedia, Isis.
[44] Wikipedia, Isis.

9.6 Ma'at

Goddess of Truth and Balance

Maat or Ma'at, at is the Goddess of concepts such as truth, balance, order, harmony, law, morality, and justice. Maat was also the Goddess who regulated the stars, seasons, and the actions of mortals and the deities who had brought an order from chaos at the moment of creation. Her ideological opposite was Isfet, who ruled over injustice, chaos, violence or to do evil.

9.7 Ra

The Sun God

Ra is the ancient Egyptian deity of the sun.

By the Fifth Dynasty in the 25th and 24th centuries BC, he was one of the most important Gods in the ancient Egyptian religion, identified primarily with the noon sun. Ra was believed to rule in all parts of the created world: the sky, the Earth, and the underworld. He was the god of the sun, order, kings, and the sky.

Ra was portrayed as a falcon and shared characteristics with the sky god Horus. The two deities were merged as Ra-Horakhty. In the New Kingdom, when the god Amun rose to prominence, he was fused with Ra into Amun-Ra.

All forms of life were believed to have been created by Ra. In some accounts, humans were created from Ra's tears and sweat; hence the Egyptians call themselves the "Cattle of Ra." In the myth of the Celestial Cow, it is recounted how humanity plotted against Ra and how he sent his

Figure 2. Ra, the Sun God

eye as the Goddess Sekhmet to punish them.[45]

Ra was the ruler of the heavens. He was the god of the sun, the bringer of light, and patron to the pharaohs. According to legend, the sun travels the skies as Ra drives his chariot through the heavens. Although he originally was associated only with the midday sun, as time went by, Ra became connected to the sun's presence all day long.

9.8 Set

Set or Seth or Sutekh

Seth is the god of deserts, storms, envy, disorder, violence, and foreigners in ancient Egyptian religion. In Ancient Greek, the god's name is given as Sēth. Seth had a positive role where he accompanies Ra on his solar boat to repel Apep, the serpent of Chaos. Seth had a vital role as a

---

[45] Wikipedia, Ra.

reconciled combatant. He was lord of the red desert land, where he was the balance to Horus's role as lord of the black soil land.[46]

In the Osiris myth, the most important Egyptian myth, Seth is portrayed as the usurper who killed and mutilated his own brother, Osiris. Osiris's wife Isis reassembled his corpse and resurrected her dead husband long enough to conceive his son and heir Horus. Horus sought revenge upon Set and the myths describe their conflicts. [47]

In ancient Egyptian astronomy, Seth was commonly associated with the planet Mercury.

---

[46] Wikipedia, Seth.
[47] Wikipedia, Seth.

A druid was a member of the high-ranking class in ancient Celtic cultures.[48]

Perhaps best remembered as religious leaders, they were also legal authorities, adjudicators, lore keepers, medical professionals, and political advisors. While the druids are reported to have been literate, they are believed to have been prevented by doctrine from recording their knowledge in written form; thus they left no written accounts of themselves. They are, however, attested in some detail by their contemporaries from other cultures, such as the Romans and the Greeks. [49]

The earliest known references to the druid's date to the fourth century BCE, and the oldest detailed description, comes from Julius Caesar's Commentarii de Bello Gallico in the '50s BCE. They were described by other Roman writers such as Cicero, Tacitus, and Pliny the Elder. Following the Roman invasion of Gaul, the druid orders were suppressed by the Roman government under the first century AD emperors Tiberius and Claudius, and had disappeared from the written record by the second century. [50]

In about 750 CE, the word druid appears in a poem by Blathmac, who wrote about Jesus, saying that he was "better than a prophet, more knowledgeable than every druid, a king who was a bishop and a complete sage." The druids appear in some of the medieval tales from Christianized Ireland, like the "Táin Bó Cúailnge," where they are largely portrayed as sorcerers who opposed the coming of Christianity. In the wake of the Celtic revival during the 18th and 19th centuries, fraternal and neopagan groups were founded based on ideas about the ancient druids, a movement known as Neo-Druidism. Many popular notions about druids, based on misconceptions of 18th century scholars, have been largely superseded by more recent study. [51]

The druids played an important part in pagan Celtic society. Julius Caesar claimed they were one of the two most important social groups in the region: nobles and organized worship and sacrifices, divination, and judicial procedure in Gaulish, British, and Irish societies. Druids were exempt from military service and from the payment of taxes, and had the power to excommunicate people from religious festivals, making them social outcasts. Two other classical writers, Diodorus Siculus and Strabo, wrote about the role of druids in Gallic society, claiming that the druids were held in such respect that if they intervened between two armies, they could stop the battle.

The Roman conquest of Britain started in AD 43 in the Reign of the Emperor Claudius and was completed by AD 87. The druids encountered by the Romans during their invasion of Gaul[52], roughly modern-day France, Luxembourg, Belgium and Switzerland. Were suppressed and gone by the start of the conquest. Although the Romans were notorious for their gladiatorial games and death that went with them, their initial problem with the druids in Britain was their use of human sacrifice in druidic rituals.

Most sacrificial victims were criminals, but if there were insufficient criminals available, innocent people were preferable. Notable means of sacrifice involved burning alive, hanging, drowning and

---

[48] Wikipedia, Druid.
[49] Wikipedia, Druid.
[50] Wikipedia, Druid.
[51] Wikipedia, Druid.
[52] Wikipedia, Gaul.

burning alive in a Wicker Man.[53] A Wicker Man was a hollow human shaped construction approximately 20–30 feet tall into which the sacrificial victims were placed and burned alive when the whicker man was set alight.

Some argue that druids in Britain did not practise human sacrifice widely until they came into contact with the Romans during the conquest. However, there have been human remains found at several druidic sites which appear to be foundational sacrifices. That is a sacrifice at the establishment/construction/consecration of the site by druids with no further human sacrifice taking place.

Druids did not write any of their rituals or lore down. This was not because they were illiterate, it was so that transmission of rituals and druidic knowledge could be controlled. Knowledge was contained in poems and verse which was learned by writing and could take years to gain full comprehension.

In Irish folklore druids serve lords and kings as high-ranking priest counselors with the gift of prophecy and other assorted mystical abilities—the best example of these possibly being Cathbad[54]. The chief druid in the court of King Conchobar mac Nessa of Ulster Cathbad was renowned for being able to tell the future. In the tale of Deirdre of the sorrows—the foremost tragic heroine of the Ulster Cycle—the druid prophesied before the court of Conchobar that Deirdre would grow up to be exquisite, but that kings and lords would go to war over her, much blood would be shed because of her, and Ulster's three greatest warriors would be forced into exile for her sake. This prophecy, ignored by the king, came true.[55]

---

[53] Wikipedia, Wickerman.
[54] Wikipedia, Cathbad.
[55] Wikipedia, Cathbad.

11 Tengrism [Mongol]

11.1 Tngri, Tengri

The Tengri religion has been recorded in Chinese chronicles from the fourth century BC onwards. Tngri was the sky god and prevailing religion of the Xiongnu, Bulgars, Huns, and possibly the Manus and Magyars people.[56] It was also the state religion of several medieval states: as: Göktürk Khaganate, Western Turkic Khaganate, Eastern Turkic Khaganate, Old Great Bulgaria, Danube Bulgaria, Volga Bulgaria, and Eastern Tourkia (Khazaria). [57]

In Tengriism, the meaning of life is found in living in harmony with the natural universe. Tengriist believers view their existence as sustained by the celestial blue sky, Tengri, the fertile Mother-Earth, and life-spirit Eje. Heaven, Earth, the spirits of nature and ancestors provide for every need and protect all humans. By living an upright and respectful life, a human being will keep his world in balance and experience prosperity, well-being and success. Shamans play an important role in restoring balance when a disaster or illness occurs.[58]

In the pantheon of Mongolian shamanism, Tngri, Tengri, or Tegri make up the highest class of divinities.

Different references describe various chief deities. The deities are divided into groups which included black and terrifying, and white or benevolent, as well as based on the points of the compass.[59]

The clan-based Mongolian society is based on a complex spiritual hierarchy.[60] They are attested too in the oldest written source in Mongolian, The Secret History of the Mongols.[61] The highest deity, Tngri, is the "supreme god of heaven" and is derived from, the primary chief deity in the religion of the early Turkic[62] and Mongolic[63] peoples, and also goes by Möngke Tngri ("Eternal Heaven") or Erketü Tngri ("Mighty Heaven"); he rules the 99 Tngri as Köke Möngke Tngri ("Blue Eternal Heaven").[64]

Several further divisions are possible, the Tngri comprises groups including the gods of the four corners, five wind gods, five gods of the entrance and five of the doors, five of the horizontal, plus many more.[65]

At the top of the hierarchy are 99 Tngri of which 55 are "white," or benevolent, and 44 terrifying or "black," There are 77 natigais or "earth mothers" plus several others. The Tngri was called upon only by leaders and great shamans and were common to all the clans. Black Tngri was invoked only by black shamans 'against evil from outside and for securing victory in war.'[66]

---

[56] Wikipedia, Xiongnu.
[57] Wikipedia, Tengrism.
[58] https://www.newworldencyclopedia.org/entry/Tengriism, TengriismNewWorldEncyclopedia.
[59] Wikipedia, Tngri.
[60] Wikipedia, Tngri.
[61] Wikipedia, TheSecretHistoryoftheMongols.
[62] Wikipedia, Turkiclanguages.
[63] Wikipedia, Mongols.
[64] Wikipedia, Tngri.
[65] Wikipedia, Tngri.
[66] Wikipedia, Tngri.

<u>Other Souls and Spirits included…</u>

- Souls of the Great Shamans: Protector-Spirits of the Clan

- Souls of the Simple Shamans: Guardian-Spirits of Localities

- The Three Spirits Accepting Supplication

<u>Division of the gods and spirits of Mongol shamanism:</u>

- White and Black deities

- Lord-Spirits of the clan

- Protector-Spirits of the clan

- Guardian-Spirits of the clan

- White Spirit of Nobles of the clan

- Black Spirits of Commoners of the clan

- Evil Spirits

Associated with Tengri is another chief deity, Qormusata Tngri, described by one scholar as the more active being and compared to the Hindu[67] god of heaven Indra[68]. Besides the 99 Tngri, there are also "seventy-seven levels of Mother Earth" and 33 other gods; the latter, like the Tngri, are ruled by Qormusata Tngri.[69]

Tngri is invoked only by the highest shamans and leaders for special occasions; they continue to be venerated especially in black shamanism. Chief among the Tngri is Qormusata Tngri and Mongke [Khan] Tngri.[70]

The Tengriist universe comprised three worlds:

- A lower or underground world,

- the middle world in which human beings lived,

- the upper spiritual world.

The lower world could be entered by a spiritual "river." The middle world connected with the upper world by a sacred World Tree. There are no official symbols of Tengriism. However the symbol of the World Tree with nine levels and four directions is common. Rituals and ceremonies were

---

[67] Wikipedia, Hinduism.
[68] Wikipedia, Indra.
[69] Wikipedia, Tngri.
[70] Wikipedia, Tngri.

typically performed on a mountaintop or by a sacred tree, places where human beings could come into contact with the spiritual world.[71]

The ancient Turks perceived Yer—Earth and Tengri—Spirit of the Sky as two complimentary aspects of a single beginning. Tengri was unknown. He was not visualized as a person, although he was said to have at least two sons. Tengri was considered being timeless and infinite, like a blue sky.

A man was born and lived in a material shell on the earth, distinct from other men; he was given a Kut—soul at birth by Tengri, who took it back when he died. Tengri was considered a father, Yer a mother. Tengri was supreme, and any supplication to Yer also included the name of Tengri.[72]

For the ancient Turks and Mongols, Tengri governed all existence on earth, determining the fate of individuals and that of entire nations and their rulers. Tengri was believed to act of his own volition, but with fairness, meting out rewards and punishments. It was believed that Tengri assisted those who revered him and who were active in trying to accomplish his will.

The term Kuk-Tengri—Blue Sky referred to a spiritual, celestial "sky," and the epithet "Kuk" (blue), when applied to an animal, such as a horse (Kuk at), ram (kuk teke), bull (kuk ugez), or deer (kuk bolan), was a reference to the animal's divine origin.

Tengri was omnipresent and was worshiped simply by lifting hands upwards and bowing low, praying for him to give good mind and health, and to help perform good deeds.
In Irk Bitig[73], Tengri is mentioned as Türük Tängrisi—God of Turks. According to many academics, at the imperial level, especially by the 12th—13th centuries, Tengrism was a monotheistic religion; most contemporary Tengrists still presents it as being monotheistic today.

Tengri differs from Siberian shamanism in that the people in power practising it were not small bands of hunter-gatherers like the Paleo Siberians but a continuous succession of pastoral, semi-sedentary khanates[74] and empires from the Xiongnu (founded 209 BC) to the Mongol Empire (13th century).[75]

Tengri developed in the eastern steppes and enjoyed more centralized and hierarchical forms of government than in the western steppe. It is more centralized and less polytheistic, less myth—intensive and more historically focused than the paganism that grew out of the western Proto-Indo-European religion. The chief god Tengri ("Heaven") is considered strikingly similar to the Indo-European sky god *Dyeus, and the structure of the reconstructed Proto-Indo-European religion is closer to that of the early Turks than to the religion of any people of Near Eastern or Mediterranean antiquity.[76]
Archeological research has revealed that the Magyar people, today known as Hungarians, worshiped Tengri until Christianity in the 10th century.

Today, Tengrism continues to exist in the distant Turko-Mongolian regions of Russia.

---

[71] https://www.newworldencyclopedia.org/entry/Tengriism, TengriismNewWorldEncyclopedia.
[72] https://www.newworldencyclopedia.org/entry/Tengriism, TengriismNewWorldEncyclopedia.
[73] Wikipedia, IrkBitig.
[74] Wikipedia, Khanate.
[75] Wikipedia, Tengrism.
[76] Wikipedia, Tengrism.

Genghis Khan and several generations of his followers were Tengrian believers and "Shaman-Kings" until his fifth-generation descendant, Uzbeg Khan, turned to Islam in the 14th century. Old Tengrist prayers have come down to us from the Secret History of the Mongols[77] (13th century).

---

[77] Wikipedia, TheSecretHistoryoftheMongols.

S hamans and Shamanesses encompassed all that is Tengri and the world order as they saw it in their animistic belief that there is energy in all things, even plants, animals, and inanimate objects.

Tengrist Shamanism[78] includes additional spirits and gods to be worshiped and visited during healing sessions.

- Umay: goddess of fertility, and often associated with the earth-mother goddesses. The word "Umay" comes from the Mongolian "Umai" which means "womb." Umay, the goddess, is the protector of children and mothers.

- Bai-Ulgen: the deity of creation. And the next most worshiped deity after Tengri. He is the god with no end and no beginning. Therefore, he always existed and never stops being. His name comes from Turkic Bay (rich) and Ulgen (magnificent). He lives in the sky above the stars, moon and sun. Bai-Ulgen is the protector of humankind against the evil deity Erlik.

- Ulgen is the other son of Bai-Ulgen and is the ruler of the upper world.

- Erklig: The powerful god of Space. He moves the stars, moons, planets, and every cosmic object. In Tengri Shamanism, Erklig is also the master of the planet Venus. Tengri's beliefs sustain that the falling stars are the hot arrows of Erklig.

- Erlik: The evil deity of the underworld. He is also the deity of death. Erlik is the first deity created by Bai-Ulgen. Erlik is known as the son of Bai-Ulgen. But Erlik became full of pride. And his actions lead to his banishment to the underworld or hell. Erlik was also present in creating humanity. He teaches humanity how to sin. Shamans often describe him as a monster with a human body but the face and teeth of a pig.

- Erlik is associated with disasters and epidemics among people or cattle, which he caused so that man would be forced to offer him a sacrifice. People were afraid to say his name and called him Kara-Name (something black) instead. Erlik had sons who helped him to rule the underground world, where there were lakes, rivers and seas. His daughters, numbering from two to nine in Turkic myths, were described as idle, sexually promiscuous temptresses. Erlik was thought to associate closely with shamans. He rarely caused evil to man, and did not control people's souls, but evil spirits from his domain would ascend to the physical road and do harm. Sacrifices were always conducted at night.

---

[78] https://spiritualgrowthguide.com/tengri-shamanism/, TengriShamanism-TheDeitiesOfTengrism-SpiritualGrowthGuide.

N ew Tengrism is a fairly "new" term. It is not an extension of Tengri, as the Mongols and Turkic tribes on the steppes knew it when Genghis Khan ruled.

The spelling "Tengrism" for the religion of the ancient Turks is found in the works of the 19th century Kazakh Russophone ethnographer Shoqan Walikhanov. The term was introduced into a wide scientific circulation in 1956 by Jean-Paul Roux and later in the 1960s as a term for English-language papers.

A revival of Tengrism has played a role in the search for native spiritual roots and Pan-Turkism ideology since the 1990s, especially, in Kyrgyzstan, Kazakhstan, Mongolia, some autonomous republics of the Russian Federation (Tatarstan, Bashkortostan, Buryatia, Yakutia, and others), among the Crimean Karaites and Crimean Tatars.[79]

After the 1908 Young Turks Revolution[80], in what the Ottoman Empire and especially the proclamation of the Republic in 1923, a nationalist ideology of Turanism and Kemalism contributed to the revival of Tengrism. Islamic censorship was abolished, which allowed an aim study of the pre-Islamic religion of the Turks. The Turkish language was purified of Arabic, Persian and other borrowings. Several figures, if they did not officially abandon Islam, but adopted Turkic names, such as Mustafa Kemal Atatürk[81] — "father of Turks" i.e., President on Modern Turkey 1923–1958, and the historian of religion and ideologist of the Kemalist regime Ziya Gökalp (Gökalp — "sky hero"). [82]

Tengrism has been advocated in intellectual circles of the Turkic nations of Central Asia (Kyrgyzstan with Kazakhstan) and Russia, Tatarstan, Bashkortostan since the dissolution of the Soviet Union during the 1990s. Still practised, it is undergoing an organized revival in Buryatia, Sakha (Yakutia), Khakassia, Tuva and other Turkic nations in Siberia. Altaian Burkhanism and Chuvash Vattisen Yaly are movements similar to Tengrism.

Tengrism has very few active adherents - 1990s, but its revival of an ethnic religion reached a larger audience in intellectual circles. Former presidents of Kazakhstan Nursultan Nazarbayev and Kyrgyzstan Askar Akayev have called Tengrism the national, "natural" religion of the Turkic peoples. So, during the 2002 trip to Khakassia, Russia, Akayev spoke out that a visit to the Yenisei River and the runic steles made up "a pilgrimage to a holy place for the Kyrgyz" just as the pilgrimage to Mecca. Presenting Islam as foreign to the Turkic peoples, as Semitic religion together with Christianity and Judaism, adherents are found primarily among the nationalistic parties of Central Asia. Tengrism may be interpreted as a Turkic version of Russian neopaganism, which is already well established. It partly similar to the new religious movements, such as New Age.[83] [84] [85]

---

[79] Wikipedia, Tengrism.
[80] Feroz Ahmad, "The Young Turk Revolution," *Journal of Contemporary History* 3, no. 3 (2016), https://doi.org/10.1177/002200946800300302.
[81] Wikipedia, MustafaKemalAtatürk.
[82] Wikipedia, Tengrism.
[83] Merriam-Webster, DefinitionofNewAge.
[84] Wikipedia, NewAge.
[85] Wikipedia, Tengrism.

Wicca, also termed Pagan Witchcraft, is a modern pagan[86] religion. Scholars of religion categories it as both a new religious movement and as part of the occultist stream of Western esotericism. It was developed in England during the first half of the 20th century and was introduced to the public in 1954 by Gerald Gardner, a retired British civil servant. Wicca draws upon a diverse set of ancient pagan and 20th-century hermetic motifs for its theological structure and ritual practices.[87]

Wicca does not believe in the existence of the Devil; therefore, it is not a Devil worshiping religion as some have described it. Wicca believes in two Gods, a female god and a male god.[88] Neither is totally good, nor totally evil, as no living being can be completely one or the other. The Gods can be called by various names, depending on every individual's cultural background. The Goddess is the representative of life, fertility, love, beauty and everything that is tied to the more feminine things. She is symbolized by the moon, because of the moon's three phases. The Goddess is known as being the Maiden Goddess, Mother Goddess, and the Crone Goddess. Two of the most popular Triple Goddesses are Isis and Hecate. [89]

The god, the Horned God to be exact, is the one who represents hunting, which is why he is horned. The horns represent the animals which were hunted and still are, to some extent. He is the protector of all wild and tame creatures. He is related to the sun. [90]

Wicca is considered a modern interpretation of pre-Christian traditions, though some involved claim a direct line to ancient practices. It may be practised by individuals or members of groups sometimes known as covens.[91]

There are some commonalities between Wicca and the environmental aspects of Druidism, and is considered the inspiration of the goddess movement in spirituality. [92]

There is great diversity among individuals and groups that practise a Wiccan religion, but many are duotheistic, worshiping both a female goddess and a male god, sometimes referred to as a Mother Goddess and a Horned God. [93]

Other Wiccan practices are atheist, pantheist, polytheist or respectful of gods and goddesses as archetypal symbols rather than as actual or supernatural beings. Rituals in Wicca often include holidays centred on phases of the moon; solar equinoxes and solstices; elements such as fire, water, earth and air; and initiation ceremonies. [94]

---

[86] Peter Jennings, *Pagan paths : a guide to wicca, druidry, asatru, shamanism and other pagan practices* (London: Rider, 2002).

[87] Wikipedia, Wicca.

[88] http://members.tripod.com/infernal_paradise/Wicca.htm, WiccanYear.

[89] http://members.tripod.com/infernal_paradise/Wicca.htm, WiccanYear.

[90] http://members.tripod.com/infernal_paradise/Wicca.htm, WiccanYear.

[91] https://www.history.com/topics/religion/wicca, Wicca.

[92] https://www.history.com/topics/religion/wicca, Wicca.

[93] https://www.history.com/topics/religion/wicca, Wicca.

[94] https://www.history.com/topics/religion/wicca, Wicca.

Wicca has no central authority figure. Its traditional core beliefs, principles and practices were originally outlined in the 1940s and 1950s by Gerald Gardner[95] and Doreen Valiente[96], both in published books and in secret written and oral teachings passed along to their initiates. There are many variations on the core structure, and the religion grows and develops. It is divided into several diverse lineages, sects and denominations, referred to as traditions, each with its own organizational structure and level of centralization. Because of its decentralized nature, there is some disagreement over what actually makes up Wicca. Some traditions, collectively referred to as British Traditional Wicca [BTW], strictly follow the initiatory lineage of Gardner and consider the term Wicca to apply only to similar traditions, but not to newer, eclectic traditions. [97]

Although pronounced differently, the Modern English term "Wicca" is derived from the Old English Wicca and wicce, the masculine and feminine term for a witch, respectively, that was used in Anglo-Saxon England[98]. By adopting it for modern usage, Wiccans were both symbolically cementing their presumed connection to the ancient, pre-Christian past, and adopting a self-designation that would be less controversial than "Witchcraft." The scholar of religion and Wiccan priestess Joanne Pearson noted that while "the words 'witch' and 'wicca' are therefore linked etymologically, they are used to emphasizing different things today." [99]

Wiccan worship of a horned god of fertility and a Mother Goddess results in many practitioners believing these deities have been worshiped since the Old Stone Age or Paleolithic or Paleolithic era, approx. 3.3 million years ago.

---

[95] Wikipedia, GeraldGardner.
[96] Wikipedia, DoreenValiente.
[97] Wikipedia, Wicca.
[98] Wikipedia, HistoryofAnglo-SaxonEngland.
[99] Wikipedia, Wicca.

The Wiccan Year[100]		
Celebration	Pronunciation and Date	Description
SAMHAN	Sow-En—Oct 31st	The first celebration of Winter, start of the Celtic New Year. A time for both beginnings and endings, through death in winter to rebirth in spring.
Yule	Yule—December 21st	Yule is the Winter Solstice, the shortest day and longest night of the year. The precise date will change from year to year. The darkest time between Samhain and Yule draws to an end as the Goddess, Mother Earth, gives birth to the Sun again.
Imbolc	EM-bowl'g—February 1st	Imbolc is the Sabbat that celebrates and honours the Goddess as the bride-to-be of the returning Sun God.
Ostara	Ostara—March 20th	Spring Equinox. Ostara is the Sabbat of Balance. The days and nights are of equal length but the Sun God is gaining more power over the darkness of Winter.
Beltane	Beltane—May 1st	As Samhain was the beginning of the cycle of Winter, Beltane marks the second major cycle of the year: Summer.
Midsummer	Midsummer—June 20th	Summer Solstice. Midsummer is the time when Father Sun reaches the highest power, Mother Earth is green and holds the promise of a bountiful harvest.
Lughnasadih	Loo-NAHS-ah August 1st	Lughnasadh is a grain harvest festival. The Goddess is honoured as the Mother who has given birth to a bounty and abundance and the God as Father of Prosperity.
Mabon	Mabon—September 22nd	Mabon is the second harvest festival on the Wheel of the Year. This Sabbat particularly celebrates the harvests of the vine, wine and apples as symbols of life renewed.

15 Ancestor Worship

The veneration of the dead, including one's ancestors, is based on love and respect for the deceased.[101]

---

[100] http://members.tripod.com/infernal_paradise/Wicca.htm, WiccanYear.
[101] Wikipedia, Venerationofthedead.

In some cultures, ancestor worship is related to beliefs that the dead have a continued existence, and may possess the ability to influence the fortune of the living. Ancestors are being able to intercede on behalf of the living, often as messengers between humans and God. Religions, such as the Eastern Orthodox and Roman Catholic Churches, venerate saints as intercessors with God; the latter also believes in prayer for departed souls in Purgatory. Other religious groups, however, consider veneration of the dead to be idolatry and a sin.[102]

Ancestors were once living beings. As a young child, I can recall sitting in my grandmother's wonderful old arm chair when she was not around. I could touch her and watch her as she cooked. She knew what I was thinking, and sometimes I knew what she thought of me and how earnest my bringing up.

As an ancestor spirt, she can understand the challenges and successes of my life. While some cultures would say her spirit, and those of my parents are there not for me to ask for favours but to do one's family duty. Others believe their ancestors need to be provided for by their descendants, and their practices include offerings of food and other provisions. While still others do not believe ancestors are aware of what their descendants do for them, but that the expression of piety is important.

Most cultures who practise ancestor veneration do not call it "ancestor worship" because of the word "worship." We go to church to worship God, Jesus Christ, or Mary Magdalene, a saint or a miraculous event. Linking this form of belief to our ancestors seems strange or wrong because in the west, they are not considered having become deities when they die.

Ancestor worship as an expression of family loyalty rather than deity worship and can be seen in simple things such as visiting a deceased relative's grave, laying flowers on a grave, praying for them on their birthday or just simply finding some time to think about them on Mother's Day or Father's Day.

Rather, the act is a way to express family duty, devotion and respect and look after ancestors in their afterlives and seek their guidance for their living descendants. Many cultures and religions have similar practices. Excluded from this are rites for the dead having no specific reference to kin, and beliefs about the dead that lack any special reference to kinship.
Asking your parents, "what would you do?" When faced with a problem could be seen as ancestor worship because we are asking for their help and guidance to sort out a difficulty we have.

"Veneration of Ancestors" to those with a Western European Christian tradition feels more appropriate, but it does not completely convey an accurate sense of what practitioners such as the Chinese and other Buddhist and Confucian-influenced societies, as well as the African and European cultures see themselves as doing. Their actions are consistent with the meaning of the word veneration in English, that is great respect or reverence caused by the dignity, wisdom, or dedication of a person.[103]

Ancestor worship is often viewed as a religious practice rather than a religion as there is seldom a priesthood attached to it and there is no formal doctrine. In most cases, ancestor worship is not the only religious practice of a society; rather, it exists as part of a more comprehensive religious system.

---

102 Wikipedia, Venerationofthedead.
103 Wikipedia, Venerationofthedead.

Death rites, including funerary and mortuary rituals, are regarded as falling within the purview of ancestor worship only when memorial rites beyond the period of death and disposition of the corpse are carried out as a regular function of a kinship group.[104]

The earliest evidence of ancestor worship in China dates to the Yangshao society, which existed in the Shaanxi Province area before spreading to parts of northern and central China during the Neolithic period - 6000 to 1000 BCE. During the Shang dynasty, 1600 - 1046 BCE, the ancestors of the royal family were thought to live in heaven within the feudal hierarchy of other spirit gods.

These ancestors, it was believed, could be contacted via a shaman. The shaman may help commune with ancestors on behalf of living family members, but it is the descendant alone that shall address his/her own forefathers to intercede in resolving family or individual conflict.

A shaman engaged in a healing ritual may contact the client's ancestors seeking help and advice in the cause and solution of the illness. The shaman may also negotiate with an ancestor who is upset about the actions of their living relatives and is causing illness or problems as a "punishment" or way to express their anger.

Advice received by the shaman from an ancestor may take them to another sprint or location in the realm they are visiting. Therefore, ancestor spirits are one form of spirit the shaman encounters when searching for answers to questions and to perform healing.

---

[104] https://www.encyclopedia.com/environment/encyclopedias-almanacs-transcripts-and-maps/ancestors-ancestor-worship, AncestorsAncestorWorship.com.

16 Animism and Paganism

Paganism is a term first used in the fourth century by early Christians for people in the Roman Empire who practised polytheism. This was because they were increasingly rural relative to the Christian population, or because they were not milites Christi—soldiers of Christ. Alternate terms in Christian texts for the same group were Hellenes, gentile, and heathen. Ritual sacrifice was an integral part of ancient Greco-Roman religion and was regarded as a sign of whether a person was pagan or Christian.[105]

Paganism was originally a pejorative and derogatory term for polytheism, implying its inferiority. Paganism has broadly connoted the "religion of the peasantry." During and after the Middle Ages, the term paganism applied to any unfamiliar religion, and the term presumed a belief in false God or Gods. Most modern pagan religions exist today. Modern or Neopaganism expresses a world view that is pantheistic, polytheistic or animistic; some are monotheistic. [106]

16.1 Polytheism

Polytheism is the worship of or belief in multiple deities, which are usually assembled into a pantheon of gods and goddesses, along with their own religions and rituals. In most religions which accept polytheism, the different gods and goddesses are representations of forces of nature or ancestral principles, and can be viewed either as autonomous or as aspects or emanations of a creator deity or transcendental absolute principle monistic theologies, which manifests immanently in nature pantheistic and pantheistic theologies. Most of the polytheistic deities of ancient religions, with the notable exceptions of the Ancient Egyptian and Hindu deities, were conceived as having physical bodies.[107]

---

[105] Wikipedia, Paganism.
[106] Wikipedia, Paganism.
[107] Wikipedia, Polytheism.

Although Westerners often use the generic term "shaman" to describe all the tribal magical practitioners of Siberia and Mongolia, they were divided into several types, categories, or classes with specific magical duties and responsibilities. Using English terminology, these included "conjurors" who summoned and controlled spirits, prophets or psychics who foresaw the future, sorcerers who practised "black magic," trance workers who travelled in spirit form to the Otherworld, healers who were experts in folk medicine and herbalism, and guides to the dead who laid out corpses and conducted funeral rites.[108]

In reality, Shame is a very spiritual person besides their other roles as healers, bonesetters, midwives and advisors.

- Bone Setter. As the description implies, their role is focused on setting bones and resolving dislocations. They also work with back pain, bowls, sores, and other skin diseases. It is often said that a bone setter can see a broken bone and an imaging device.

- Midwife. The Shaman midwife inherited her power from the maternal line of familial descent. As well as ensuring that babies entered this world safely in a physical sense, she was also responsible for their spiritual protection from evil influences during birth and their well-being as children. In this sense she took on the role of a human faerie godmother. Immediately after a birth the shaman-midwife cut the umbilical cord and then purified the newborn baby with salt water and fire. Any (female only) witnesses to the birth could only be present if they had first been ritually purified by the midwife with fire and water. During the first few weeks of a baby's life, it was very important that the proper rituals were performed to protect the child until its spirit was fully established in the material world. If they were not performed properly, then the baby's spirit might return whence it had come. These essential rites were the responsibility of the shaman midwife and her assistants.[109]

- Shaman Smith. One of the most important and respected types of magical practitioners was the Shaman Smith. In all cultures all over the world from Europe to Africa, the Smith took a central role in tribal society and was regarded as a powerful magician or sorcerer because of his mastery over fire and skill in working with metal. In Siberia, the shaman smiths made and magically consecrated the ritual metal objects used by other shamans. They were only chosen by the spirits and instead of a drum; they used their anvils to communicate with the spiritual realm. Healer and Guide. [110]

- Shaman Assistant. The role has various duties, ranging from warming the drums by the fire, over helping with the equipment up to drumming, which make up some of the most common duties. Shaman assistants are usually people who are very spiritual but have never

---

[108] https://www.newdawnmagazine.com/articles/secrets-of-siberian-shamanism, SecretsofSiberianShamanism.
[109] https://www.newdawnmagazine.com/articles/secrets-of-siberian-shamanism, SecretsofSiberianShamanism.
[110] https://www.newdawnmagazine.com/articles/secrets-of-siberian-shamanism, SecretsofSiberianShamanism.

had a specific calling. They do not wear specialized regalia, but often the shaman they work with gives them a protective talisman as a gift.[111]

17.1 Healer and Guide

The shaman is a healer. This is their principal role in the tribe, the community.

They have access to, and influence in, the world of benevolent and malevolent spirits, who typically enter a trance state during a ritual, and practices divination and healing.

Soul journeying to understand what and why a person was ill and journeying to spirits that will help return health to the physical person is their primary and most essential role.

Mongol shamanism had ninety-nine deities:

- Fifty-five deities were White, i.e., Beneficent for humanity.
- Forty-four were Black, i.e., Terribles to all the evildoers of humanity and to the enemies of the Mongol Nation.

They are the national gods of Mongol Shamanism. No commoner of any Mongol clan dared embarrass them with his insubstantial bagatelle, since they were the Spirits of Ancestors of every clan, the souls of dead chieftains, shamans and Shamanesses who during their life had devoted themselves to satisfying the members of clans and who in the World of Spirits should solve the difficulties in the life of the members of their clans, commoners and nobles and even serfs.

Minor spirits of a clan's ancestors divided into several classes. The largest among them were the class of the souls of the clans' chieftains, introduced after their death by a special solemn shamanist rite to the communion of Clan Ancestors and thus becoming members of the communion and of the Benevolent Lord-Spirits who played a very important role in the life of a clan and its members.

Black shamanism is a kind of shamanism practised in Mongolia and Siberia. It is specifically opposed to yellow shamanism, which incorporates rituals and traditions from Buddhism. Black Shamans are usually perceived as working with evil spirits, while white Shamans are inin spirits of the upper world.

Other Souls and Spirits included…

- Souls of the Great Shamans: Protector-Spirits of the Clan
- Souls of the Simple Shamans: Guardian-Spirits of Localities
- The Three Spirits Accepting Supplication

<u>Division of the gods and spirits of Mongol shamanism:</u>

White and Black deities
Lord-Spirits of the clan

---

[111] http://www.face-music.ch/bi_bid/historyoftengerism.html, ShamanismTengerisminMongoliainEnglish.

Protector-Spirits of the clan
Guardian-Spirits of the clan
White Spirits of Nobles of the clan
Black Spirits of Commoners of the clan
Evil Spirits

Chinggis Khan, or Genghis Khan, the renowned Mongolian leader, practised Black Shamanism, though he himself was not a shaman.

The banner at the head of the Mongol Armies that subjugated China and got as far as eastern Europe was black. But this should not be confused with Chinggis Khan and his practice of Black Shamanism. A tribe would have black and white banners in the centre of their camp.

The banners were each guarded together with white and black Lord Spirits of the Clan. Nobles of the clan would escort the banners during ceremonies and feasts.

In battle, the black banner was believed to bring victory over Mongol enemies while the white banner remained in camp.

17.2 Oracle

Shaman was astrologers and oracles. Everyone, especially tribal leaders, wants to know what the future will bring. Will it bring war? Will they be successful in the struggle? Will crops and animal husbandry be successful? Will the tribe merge with another through marriage?

The history of the shaman in this role goes back into the very remote past, before Buddhism in Tibet in the seventh century.

Historically, these oracles, divination and Astrology were a feature of Bon in pre-Buddhist Tibet. The Bon cosmology was divided into three worlds.

- The upper world of the gods.
- An intermediate world of spirits, of subtle beings.
- The solid or physical world we know as the earth.

Bon also held the spirit or soul of the individual, which was a world or realm of energy which humans can contact. For example, humans can connect with physical things such as food, a chair and other people. On the spiritual level, they can connect at the psychic level with other spirits and those on the different levels, such as the first and second.

When Buddhists brought Buddhist Dharma to Tibet, they could include the Bon world view into their own because Buddhism holds the view. The Buddhist world exists in three parts: one solid, one psychic, and one mental.

The change happened when the famous Tantric master Guru Padmasambhava came to Tibet and tamed the subtle world—the deities of the Bonpos—and bound them under oath to obey and defend the Buddhist teaching. He made these powers, which we can call deities, protectors of the Buddhist faith and of Buddhist practitioners. They became Cho sung, protectors of the Dharma.

According to Tibetan tradition, he tamed these beings through the powerful invocation of mantras, powerful spells, which bound them to obey those who held the power of these spells. Guru Padmasambhava tamed these beings. He made them protectors of the Dharma and obliged or convinced them to help practitioners of Buddha Dharma by communicating, giving advice, foretelling the future and even healing people.

The deities are sentient beings. They are beings, just like people or animals and anyone else, but without a body. They also have a mind or spirit, and a voice. Without a body, they cannot communicate with those who communicate on a bodily level. So, they are samsaric beings.

Samsara is the term for the everlasting cycle of being. It is the cycle of becoming and passing away, or the cycle of rebirths in the Indian religions of Hinduism, Buddhism, and Jainism.

They are not higher gods, as we would understand the great gods of India or Tibet. They are gods linked to the land, mountains, lakes and to the geographical features. We could, in a way to say that mountains and lakes are their bodily aspect. So, they are the subtle aspect: the speech and mind aspect of mountains, valleys, rivers and lakes, especially mountains and lakes.

17.3 Continuity

They were the spiritual leader of a group or tribe. The belief and practice of Shamanism incorporate a range of beliefs, customs, ceremonies and rituals regarding communication with the spiritual world in which their religious leader, the Shaman, enters supernatural realms particularly when the tribe is facing adversity or need to get solutions to problems afflicting the community including sickness.

They provided continuity to the tribe and a reliable connection to the spirit world. In this way, they were a communicator from the human physical world to the spirit world and back again.
They were an educator of people about the spirit world and about medicines and herbs and natural healing solutions. They kept the tribal stories, myths and essential tribal wisdom that made the tribe they belonged to different from another.

They understood and passed down understanding of trance states, how to induce them and how to control them. Their clothing, symbolic regalia and objects were passed down to enrich subsequent generations of shaman.

They are the keepers of tradition, ancient texts, books, and scripts and the way things should be done. Songs, dances, music, and observance are also carried forward from the shaman to shamans within the tribe.

Shamans usually have expert knowledge of medicinal plants native to their area, and an herbal treatment is often prescribed. It is believed shamans learn directly from the plants, harnessing their effects and healing properties, after obtaining permission from the indwelling or patron spirits.

The chieftains and nobles may change, but the shaman remains.

17.4 Protector

One of a shaman's major functions is to protect individuals from hostile supernatural influences.

The shaman may act as a psychopomp, conducting the spirits of individuals who have just died to the proper refuge for dead spirits.

Psychopomp literally means "guide of souls" are creatures, spirits, angels, or deities in many religions whose responsibility is to escort newly deceased souls from Earth to the afterlife. They do not judge the deceased, but simply to guide them. Appearing frequently on funerary art, psychopomps have been depicted at different times and in different cultures as anthropomorphic entities, horses, deer, dogs, whip-poor-wills, ravens, crows, vultures, owls, sparrows and cuckoos. When seen as birds, they are often seen in vast masses, waiting outside the home of the dying.

17.5   Other Traditions of Shaman Selection

Banjhakri [112] and Banjhākrini[113] are shamanic deities in the tradition of the Kirati people of Nepal[114]. They are a couple, and possibly different aspects of the same being. They are supernatural shamans of the forest. In the Nepali language, ban means "wilderness," jhākri means "shaman," and Jhākrini means "shamaness." Banjhākrini is also known as Lemlemey.
Banjhākri is a short, wild, simian trickster who is a descendant of the Sun. His ears are large and his feet point backward. Long, matted hair covers his entire body, except for his face and palms, and he plays a golden dhyāngro. The dhyangro is the frame drum played by Nepali jhākri.

Banjhākri finds human children who have the potential to be great shamans and takes them back to his cave for training.

The abductee is taught about the forest, spirits, life, death, and healing. Taught in this way, when the abductee was returned to their home, their village, their community, after a few days, they were more powerful than any shaman taught by a human. They are prototypical models for becoming a shaman in Nepal and, so to speak, a mark of distinction and an epithet of supernatural potency and unofficial status. The abductee may be taken again for further training. The Banjhākri may also appear in dreams to continue teaching.

If the abductee were found to have physical problems, scars, or not pure of heart, or if they failed the initiation ceremony at the end of their stay, or had been disobedient, they would be thrown out of the Banjhakri camp and risked being captured by his ferocious and cannibalistic mate, the Banjhakrini who would kill them with her gold cycle and eat their bodies.

In all the stories about the Banjhakri, they are the teacher, the guide, the instructor, the leader, the mentor, but now he wanted to learn. They teach using a combination of telepathy and a secret language the initiate learns.

Like the yeti, Banjhakri and Banjhakrini can be seen in our world, and not just in the spirit world. However, only powerful shamans can see them. Although both Banjhakri and yeti are apelike, yeti is taller than humans, whereas Banjhakri is only about 1–1.5 m (3–5 feet) tall. Both have fur covering their entire body except for their hands and their face. Their feet face backwards. This means if tracks are found, the trackers are inevitably going in the wrong direction if they follow the impressions, believing them to be normal human feet. The yeti lives in the high mountain pass and

---

112 Wikipedia, BanjhakriandBanjhakrini.
113 Wikipedia, BanjhakriandBanjhakrini.

are teachers of yogis and others that seek the peace and energy of high mountains and live there, in caves.

The Banjhakri are the masters of Liminality. They stand at the juncture of two realities, in between categories and boundaries. They are physical and spiritual. Human and animal, beings of dreams and of reality. They are the masters in a numinous unbounded space where everything is backwards, opposite, and dangerous. They are the neophytes' guides through the dark night before initiatory rebirth.

We are used to seeing and thinking of shamans in their traditional cultures. But there is a shaman alive and well today and they walk, talk, and dress in how to fit in completely with the societies in which they live.

A person visiting a traditional shaman, in a traditional culture, may not think twice about a shaman dressing in a bearskin to call on and work with a helping spirit who is a bear. In modern western culture, that would not be acceptable. A modern shaman may wear a bear claw on a chain or cord under their shirt instead. The claw would not be seen by anyone present, but the effect would be the same during the ceremony. And there is a shaman who has such a relationship with their helping spirits that even a bear claw is not required.

A few years ago, I developed an intense pain in my back and had difficulty breathing. An ambulance took me to the hospital where I spent the rest of the day and a night in the Emergency Room. Lying on the bed, surround by curtains, I could only hear the voices and words of the other patients, doctors, and nurses. There was nothing to see. It seemed as if they were from another world.

In the spaces next to me, patients would come and go. The space next to me suddenly was filled with violent words spoken with terrible energy and the sounds of metal restraints jangling against the fastening points of the bed. The patient had been strapped and chained to their bed. They were confined and in pain. I heard it all. It went on for hours. Finally, the diagnosis was that a family doctor had changed the calming meditation prescribed by the hospital and the change was not a pleasant change.

After a few hours on different medications, the patient was quietened, and they disappeared to somewhere else in the hospital and a special cleaning staff arrived to wipe down and sanitize the space the patient had occupied.

Then, in the distance, the sound of a caring relative to an elderly relative, their father whom they loved very much. Whatever the cause, the elderly relative had been fitted with a diaper and the vice was encouraging him to use the diaper, but the fates resisted. Throughout their life they did as they had been brought up to do, use a toilet. Lying or sitting and simply peeing were not the way they had lived their life. The caring relative calmly and repeatedly affirmed that now was different, life was different, and so was their existence.

Then, a slight break in the curtains. I could see out. I could see an elderly man and his relatives. He had just arrived and seemed to be quite lively, but as the hours passed, the life essence of him drained away. At the point I left the ER, he was unresponsive and several conferences with doctors had come and gone. Now that I look at it, his soul was ready to leave, but his physical container, his body, was still holding on with its autonomic processes.

I have always been aware of my guides, one in particular. She has looked after and helped me many times and we have a strong relationship.

At 1 a.m. a "white alert" was announced over the intercom. Sounds of screaming, swearing and smashing of equipment and doors banging raged through the ER. A patient with a mental disorder had sided step their attendant and was roaming the ER. The sounds would be distant one moment and almost next to my small curtained space the next. It seemed to be a soul in torment, tormented by a dark energy that would eventually destroy the physical container.

I called on my guides and with all my heart affirmed by adherence to "being a soul, a spirit of light, and love," today I would say I am a white shaman. As I affirmed my intention repeatedly, the tortured voice became more distant, and was gone.

A flurry of activity with doctors followed. They had diagnosed a blood clot on the back of one of my lungs. I was released several hours later with a course of medication and follow-up tests to be done.

It was a month after this experience that a new guide appeared, a Tibetan White Shaman. She had been born in AD 521. She would lead me through the induction as a White Shaman, and together with my Reiki guides, would provide shamanic energy and experience to healing sessions.

A very modern, shamanic initiation crisis which differs from traditional initiatory crisis of the future shaman is usually shown by involuntary shaking, induced by the Spirits in some form or other. This state is also called the "shamanic illness." The shamanistic initiatory crisis functions as an—involuntary—rite of passage for the future shaman, and it involves both a more-or-less serious physical illness and/or a psychological crisis. This state is well attested across all shamanic regions. Next to illness, the shaman-to-be may be struck by lightning and may dream of thunder, or may have a near-death experience.

18 Shamanic Soul

T he Catholic theologian Thomas Aquinas attributed "soul" to all organisms but argued that only human souls are immortal. Other religions, most notably Hinduism and Jainism, hold that all living things from the smallest bacterium to the largest of mammals are the souls themselves and have their physical representative, the body, in the world. The actual self is the soul. The body is simply a mechanism to experience the karma of that life. Thus, if we see a tiger, then there is a self-conscious identity or soul living in it, and a physical representative of the whole body of the tiger, which is observable in the world. Some teach that even non-biological entities, such as rivers and mountains, possess souls. This belief is called animism.

Animism is a major part of the shamanic world view and an understanding of what this world represents. Shamans often work by being able to reach a different level of consciousness or awareness that allows them to speak to the spirits of the natural world, who can then provide them with knowledge and information. Shamanism often relies pretty heavily on animistic ideas with most shamanistic practices, but not all but animism can exist without shamanism.

Your soul lives inside your body in the physical world, but it also lives in the Soul World at the same time. Everyone and everything are in the Soul World, because everyone and everything has a soul.

The soul is the principle of life, feeling, thought, and action in humans. In some religions, it is believed that when the person dies, although their body is no longer alive, their spirit or soul moves on to another world. The soul in religion is needed for reincarnation, which is clear in Hinduism and Buddhism, where, when we die, our souls come back to take over the body of any living matter. Souls are not only clear in religion and philosophy.

18.1 Shamanism and Animism

Shamans have visions and perform various deeds during a trance and it is believed they have the power to control spirits in the body. They may leave normal existence and travel or fly to other worlds. Manchu-Tungus nomads of Siberia and northern China language, Shaman means "agitated or frenzied people."

Shamans are bridges between their communities and the spiritual world. During trances, which are induced during a ritual, shaman seek spirits to help cure illnesses, bring about pleasant weather, predict the future, or communicate with deceased ancestors.

Animism attributes a distinct spiritual essence or soul to objects, places and creatures all possess a distinct spiritual essence and is perceived to be in all things—animals, plants, rocks, rivers, weather systems, human handiwork and perhaps even words—as animated and alive. Animism is used in the anthropology of religion as a term for the belief system of many indigenous peoples, especially in contrast to the relatively more recent development of organized religions.[115]

There are places on earth where sacred power is concentrated. Those places are held sacred and where communication with the spirit world takes place. It is a belief in a supernatural power that organizes and animates the material universe and that ancestors watch over the living from the spirit world.

---

[115] Wikipedia, Animism.

Modern Abrahamic organized religions have an animistic fixation with holy land, holy places, or holy buildings is defined as animism but rarely called that. The sacredness of those places, where certain sacred events took place, is closely linked to and recorded to stories in the Bible.

The fervour of the religion's membership in keeping those places for its own membership is sectarian in its desire to segregate them for use by their own religion. Outsiders are excluded and maybe harmed, or even killed. The hot spot that shows isolationism, extreme nationalism, ethnocentrism, can be found in the Middle East today, particularly the "Holy Land."

18.2 Bon Sarma

Often referred to as New Bon, this is an eclectic tradition combining elements of Indian Buddhism and Yungdrung Bon, which appeared in the eighth century AD and is still very popular in eastern Tibet, particularly in Kham.

18.3 Mixed Bon

This refers to the wide range of tribal traditions practised in the borderlands surrounding Tibet and the Himalayas in which Prehistoric Bon, Yungdrung Bon and various other elements mingle in various proportions.

18.4 Bo Murgel

The Bo Murgel belief system of Mongolia and Buryatia—thousands of miles from Tibet—has many features in common with Tibetan Bon, not least of which is its name, Bo—pronounced like "boar" with a double "oar" sound.

18.5 Dzogchen?

Dzogchen, or "Great Perfection," it is a tradition of teachings in Tibetan Buddhism aimed at discovering and continuing in the natural primordial state of being. It is a central teaching of the Yungdrung-Bon tradition and in the Nyingma school of Tibetan Buddhism. In these traditions, Dzogchen is the highest and most definitive path of the nine vehicles to liberation. According to this terma, Dzogchen originated with the founder of the Bon tradition, Tonpa Shenrab.

19 Soul

The word "soul" can refer to the Spirit of God. Or, if the person speaking to me does not want to refer to "God," just "Spirit." It exists in each individual, it is ever-existing, ever-conscious, ever-new bliss.

Identification of the soul with the physical body becomes the nature of the individual. References to "spiritual progress" or "soul evolution" use this definition, because the soul that is aware of its true identity as part of God is already perfect. Souls only develop or progress in the sense that they go from identifying with their physical bodies to identifying with God. This can also be called the ego.

19.1 Dictionary Definition

- The physical structure and material substance of an animal or plant, living or dead [116]

Merriam-Webster Dictionary[117]

- the immaterial essence, animating principle, or actuating cause of an individual life

- the spiritual principle embodied in human beings, all rational and spiritual beings, or the universe

- Capitalized, Christian Science: GOD sense

- a person's total self

- an active or essential part

- of a moving spirit: LEADER

- the moral and emotional nature of human beings

- the quality that arouses emotion and sentiment

- spiritual or moral force: FERVOUR

19.2 Etymology

In Modern English, the word "soul" is derived from Old English sáwol, sáwel, was first attested in the 8th century poem Beowulf v. 2820 and in the Vespasian Psalter 77.50. It is cognate with other German and Baltic terms for the same idea, including Gothic saiwala, Old High German sêula, sêla, Old Saxon sêola, Old Low Franconian sêla, sîla, Old Norse sála and Lithuanian siela. Deeper etymology of the Germanic word is unclear.[118]

---

[116] Dictionary.com, DefinitionofBodyatDictionary.com.
[117] Merriam-Webster Dictionary, DefinitionofSoulbyMerriam-Webster.
[118] Wikipedia, Soul.

The original concept behind the Germanic root is thought to mean "coming from or belonging to the sea (or lake)," because of the Germanic and pre-Celtic belief in souls emerging from and returning to sacred lakes, Old Saxon sêola (soul) compared to Old Saxon sêo (sea). [119]

In the Tibetan world view, there is no destructive death at the end of life as it is in the west. Instead, there is reincarnation, rebirth, and transition into a new life. What we do in this life, the good and bad deeds, or Karma influence the rebirth of our soul and how it will continue to seek enlightenment.

The soul[120] in many religious, philosophical, and mythological traditions, is the incorporeal[121] essence, the nonmaterial form of a living being. Soul or psyche comprises the mental abilities of a living being: reason, character, feeling, consciousness, memory, perception, thinking, etc. Depending on the philosophical system, a soul may be mortal or immortal.

19.3 Incorporeal Essence

The soul includes other forms of incorporeal essence. It includes our emotions, our will to do something, or not. Our thoughts and our feelings. It is through our soul that we sense hurt and suffering and pleasure and enjoyment. Our soul experiences the energy and drive, or discouragement of external stimulus and how we respond to it.

When we collect all these incorporeal reactions to stimulus, we come to life and others around us, human or animal react to us. Some people have good relations with other humans and animals, some do not. This outward expression of the soul becomes what we and others describe as our personality.

To a great extent, the expression of our personality is reinforced by repeated, similar reactions from those around us. External shocks and changes can change our personality. Sudden loss of a loved one, human or animal can be so fundamental that other aspects of our soul come to the surface that had previously not had expression.

19.4 Human Body

The human body is the material and physical structure of a human being. It is composed of many cells that together create tissues and, subsequently, organ systems. They ensure homeostasis and the viability of the human body. [122]

It comprises a head, neck, trunk (which includes the thorax and abdomen), arms and hands, legs and feet. [123]

The study of the human body involves anatomy, physiology, histology, and embryology. The body varies anatomically in-known ways. Physiology focuses on the systems and organs of the human

---

[119] Wikipedia, Soul.
[120] Wikipedia, Soul.
[121] Dictionary.com, Incorporeal.
[122] Wikipedia, Humanbody.
[123] Wikipedia, Humanbody.

body and their functions. Many systems and mechanisms interact in order to maintain homeostasis, with safe levels of substances such as sugar and oxygen in the blood. [124]

The body is studied by health professionals, physiologists, anatomists, and by artists to assist them in their work.[125]

It is the physical entity we interact with, on the subway, in the grocery store, at work, in love, or when we are in conflict.

The physical body is what we find attractive in a man or woman until we know the person better. It is the physical body that creates limitations, such as being confined to a wheelchair, and it grants gifts, such as being artistic or proficient and admired in sports. These gifts and limitations are part of the boundary to the learning experience of the soul and in which the spirit must work.

19.5 Other Bodies

Human beings are not the only physical beings that have a body. Animals, plants and cells also have bodies.

Animals are multicellular eukaryotic organisms that from the biological kingdom Animalia. With few exceptions, animals consume organic material, breathe oxygen, can move, can reproduce sexually, and grow from a hollow sphere of cells, the blastula, during embryonic development. Over 1.5 million living animal species have been described—of which around 1 million are insects—but it has been estimated there are over 7 million animal species in total. Animals range from 8.5 millionths of a meter to 33.6 m (110 ft). They have complex interactions with each other and their environments, forming intricate food webs. The kingdom Animalia includes humans, but in colloquial use the term animal often refers only to non-human animals. The scientific study of animals is known as zoology.[126]

When we consider the cellular world, cellular respiration[127] is a guide as to the activity in the cell and the world within and without the cell and the life process taking place in it which is a mirror of what is taking place in human and animal bodies.

The body is a complex organization of cells, bones, and connective tissues which take together inhabit physical space, whether alive or dead, even when cremated. The body's ashes take up space. If you reach out with your index finger, you can touch your body and that of other human beings and animals and you can use tools such as microscopes to study other life forms.

19.6 Spirit

What we call a Spirit[128] [129] [130] is also incorporeal. If the soul exists within us and is gathering experience through lifetime after lifetime, then in each life it is the spirit that gives expression to the

---

[124] Wikipedia, Humanbody.
[125] Wikipedia, Humanbody.
[126] Wikipedia, Animal.
[127] Wikipedia, Cellularrespiration.
[128] Wikipedia, Spirit.
[129] Dictionary.com, SpiritDefinitionofSpirit.
[130] Longman Dictionary of Contemporary English, spiritmeaningofspirit.

soul's gained knowledge and our thoughts and mental capabilities. It expresses personality, knowledge, and wisdom. It is what moves our body.

The spirit world of the shamans is not much different from the physical world. Spirits are in everything and everywhere. Spirits have physical bodies; they can fly and travel anywhere with tremendous speed and see and sense things over great distances or in the past or future. Westerners explain such phenomena with the term's telepathy or psychic abilities, talents to sense things using the abilities of the spirits which inhabit human beings. Shamans use spirits during their rituals, to fly to other places or sense things far away or in spirit form through the aid of their Utha (Heaven power) and other spirit helpers or Ongons.[131]

Because a person's soul is a combination of all that it experienced before in previous lives, plus our logic, thoughts, emotions and experiences in this life which are driven by the spirit, that spirt cannot continue after the body's physical death. Its role was to help the soul experience a lifetime of physical existence. At the moment of death, when the soul leaves the corporeal body to be reincarnated, the spirit's work is complete, and it does not continue.

19.7 Atman—Hinduism

Atman is a Sanskrit word that means inner self, spirit, or soul. In Hindu philosophy, especially in the Vedanta school of Hinduism, Atman is the first principle, the true self of an individual beyond identification with phenomena, the essence of an individual. In order to attain liberation (moksha), a human being must gain self-knowledge, which is to realize that one's true self is identical to the transcendent self-Brahman.

The six orthodox schools of Hinduism believe that there is Atman (soul, self) in every being. This is a major point of difference with the Buddhist doctrine of Anatta, which holds that there is no unchanging soul or self.

19.8 Theological Soul

Soul and the spirit are the two primary immaterial parts that Scripture ascribes to humanity.[132] The word spirit refers only to the immaterial facet of humanity. Human beings have a spirit, but we are not spirits. However, the word's soul, and spirit, are often used interchangeably, the primary distinction between soul and spirit is that in men and women the soul has animate life, or is the seat of the senses, desires, affections, and appetites.

The soul, in many religious, philosophical, and mythological traditions, is the ethereal essence of a living being. The soul or psyche comprises the mental abilities of a living being: reason, character, feeling, consciousness, memory, perception, thinking, etc. Depending on the philosophical system, a soul can either be mortal or immortal.[133] The soul, is alive, physically and eternally. The spirit can be alive, as with believers (1 Peter 3:18), or dead as unbelievers are (Colossians 2:13; Ephesians 2:4-5).

Believers in Jesus Christ and his role in salvation respond to the things that come from the Spirit of God, understanding and discerning them spiritually. The spirit allows us to connect, or not, with

---

[131] http://www.face-music.ch/bi_bid/historyoftengerism.html, ShamanismTengerisminMongoliainEnglish.
[132] GotQuestions.org, Whatisthedifferencebetweenthesoulandspiritofman?.
[133] Wikipedia, Soul.

God. Our spirits relate to His Spirit, either accepting his promptings and conviction, proving that we belong to him (Romans 8:16) or resisting him and proving that we do not have spiritual life (Acts 7:51).

The spirit is the element in humanity that gives us the ability to have an intimate relationship with God. Whenever the word spirit is used, it refers to the immaterial part of humanity that "connects" with God, who himself is spirit (John 4:24).

Judaism and Christianity teach that only human beings have immortal souls although immortality is disputed within Judaism and the concept of immortality may have been influenced by Plato.

The "origin of the soul" has provided a vexing question in Christianity. The major theories put forward include soul creationism, traducianism, and pre-existence. According to soul creationism, God creates each individual soul created directly, either at the moment of conception or some later time. According to traducianism, the soul comes from the parents by natural generation. According to the pre-existence theory, the soul exists before the moment of conception. There have been differing thoughts regarding whether human embryos have souls from conception, or whether there is a point between conception and birth where the fetus gains a soul, consciousness, and/or personhood. Stances in this question might play a role in judgments on the morality of abortion.[134]

The most basic meaning of "soul" is "life," there is no distinction whether it refers to physical or eternal life. Jesus asks what it profits a man to gain the entire world and lose his soul, referring to his eternal life (Matthew 16:26). Both Old and New Testaments reiterate we are to love God completely, with the whole "soul" which refers to everything that is in us that makes us alive (Deuteronomy 6:4-5; Mark 12:30). Whenever the word "soul" is used, it can refer to the whole person, whether physically alive or in the afterlife.

The soul is our source of absolute uniqueness, a place within that connects you not only to your own value and essence, but to the value and essence of every other living being. This is limiting. We will get back to that later.

19.9   Where Is the Soul in the Physical Body?

Debate on "where" the soul is in a physical body is large and disruptive discussion topic. Mostly because we do not have a suitable definition by which to recognize the soul if we are lucky enough or astute enough to find it!

- Descartes: The pineal gland is a tiny organ in the centre of the brain that played an important role in Descartes's philosophy. He regarded it as the principal seat of the soul and the place in which all our thoughts are formed.[135]

- Leonardo da Vinci used his experience in anatomy to hypothesize that the soul was in the optic chiasm, near the third ventricle of the brain. His views were supported by observations of change in perception following disturbances to that area of the brain.[136]

---

[134] Wikipedia, Soul.
[135] Stanford Encyclopedia of Philosophy, DescartesandthePinealGland.
[136] Wikipeda, Historyofthelocationofthesoul.

- Aristotle in De Anima (On the Soul) suggests that the organs of the body are required for the soul to interact with. Unlike Plato, Aristotle believed the soul's existence was not separate from the human body; thus the soul could not be immortal. Similarly, to Plato, however, Aristotle believed the soul is composed of three parts: the vegetative, sensitive, and rational. Growth and reproduction result from the vegetative soul, and is found in all organisms. The sensitive soul, however, allows for sensation and movement in humans and animals. The third, the rational, is exclusive to humans, and allows for rational thought.[137]

19.10 Ensoulment

After considering "where" the soul can be found in the body, how does it get there, when does it arrive?

In religion, ensoulment is the moment at which a human being gains a soul.[138] [139] Some religions say that a soul is newly created within a developing child and others, especially in religions that believe in reincarnation[140], that the soul is pre-existing and added at a particular stage of development.

In the time of Aristotle, it was widely believed that the human soul entered the forming body at 40 days (male embryos) or 90 days (female embryos), and quickening showed a soul. Other religious views are that ensoulment happens at the moment of conception; or when the child takes the first breath after being born; at the formation of the nervous system and brain; at the first brain activity (e.g., heartbeat); or, when the fetus can survive independently of the uterus (viability).[141]

The concept is closely related to debates on the morality of abortion and the morality of contraception. Religious beliefs that human life has an innate sacredness to it have motivated many statements by spiritual leaders of various traditions over the years. However, the three matters are not exactly parallel, given that various figures have argued that some kind of life without a soul, in various contexts, still has a moral worth that must be considered. [142]

---

[137] Wikipeda, Historyofthelocationofthesoul.
[138] Wikipedia, Ensoulment.
[139] https://en.wikipedia.org/wiki/The_City_of_God, TheCityofGod.
[140] http://healerofheartsandminds.com, Reincarnation,PastLives,SufferingandtheBible,AShaman'sViews.
[141] Wikipedia, Ensoulment.
[142] Wikipedia, Ensoulment.

20   Black, White and Yellow Shaman

Shamans are the preeminent healers of premodern societies. Their roles as healers include medical and psychiatric functions, addressing physical disease and a variety of psychological conditions. Shamanism provides mechanisms for inducing healing through systemic psychological integration using ritual, symbols, and ASC. Shamans' practices represent the evolution of a "holistic imperative," a drive toward more integrated levels of consciousness.[143]

Shamanic traditions produce integrative responses that synchronize divergent aspects of human cognition and identity through several mechanisms, including:

- using ASC, ritual, and symbols to activate synchronizing brain processes
- the stimulation of processes of lower-brain structures and subconscious aspects of personality and self
- Incorporating people into community rituals that strengthen social support and identity. These therapeutic processes still have relevance in the modern world, as evidenced by the modern resuscitation of the ancient shamanic practices.[144]

In the beginning … there were only two types of shamans, "black" and "white." Applying the terms white and black to shamans is often a result of the perspective from which you apply the labels. Many such decisions about labels were and still are made from a Judo-Christian viewpoint rather than the indigenous people who have existed with shaman for millennia.

White shaman refers to those who deliver "good" aims to help or heal, while black shaman refers to those who have negative or "evil" aims to hurt or even kill the victims. As Buddhism arrived in Tibet and the Mongolian steppe, a third type appeared, the "yellow shaman."

---

[143] Encyclopedia.com, Shamans.
[144] Encyclopedia.com, Shamans.

Although white and black shamans sometimes overlapped, black shamans were regarded as the most powerful and also referred to as "warrior shamans" because they battled evil forces, travelled to the underworld and were consulted as military advisors. In wartime, their role was to motivate the soldiers and population in order, hopefully, to secure victory for their own side. It was Black shamans that went on campaign with the Mongol armies, or with the tribal forces when battling other tribes. Black Shaman got their power from the North, possibly the North Pole or the North Star and could be easily identified as they always wore black robes with very little decoration. The primary function of the black shaman was to deal with demons and the dark gods on behalf of their clients. In this role they were hired to curse their enemies and blight their crops and livestock.[145]

In peacetime they acted as diplomats, political advisors and emissaries and they oversaw the preparation and signing of treaties with the appropriate magical rites. Black shamans were feared, even after their deaths. In the 19th century, when a famous one died; she was placed in a coffin made from the "unclean" wood of an aspen. Her corpse was then nailed down with aspen stakes so she could not become a "night walker" and haunt the living.[146]

Black Shamans maybe malevolent sorcerers who masquerade as real shamans and who entice tourists to drink ayahuasca in their presence. Shamans believe one purpose for this is to steal the drinker's energy or power, of which they believe every person has a limited stockpile.[147]

During their initiation, a Buryat[148], Black Shaman must take ninety-nine oaths which prevents them from causing any kind of harm. She said; it was prohibited to endanger human life, put obstacles in people's way and quarrel, but they have to help all the living creatures.[149] Black shaman from other ethnic groups and tribes are not obliged to take such oaths.

The costume worn by a Black shaman is considered their armour against attacks by black or harmful spirits. The costume includes miniature iron weapons believed to have been forged by Damdin Dorlig, the patron deity of blacksmiths, who is also regarded as an armourer of shamans.

The longer a Black Shaman has practised, the more and varied will be iron weapons they will have on their costume. This is because the more experienced Shaman will encounter stronger and more varied dark spirits in their work to expel dark spirits from a client.

---

[145] https://www.newdawnmagazine.com/articles/secrets-of-siberian-shamanism, SecretsofSiberianShamanism.
[146] https://www.newdawnmagazine.com/articles/secrets-of-siberian-shamanism, SecretsofSiberianShamanism.
147 http://situgen.blogspot.com/search/label/shaman%27s%20costume, shaman'scostume.
148 https://en.wikipedia.org/wiki/Buryatia, Buryatia.
149 http://situgen.blogspot.com/search/label/shaman%27s%20costume, shaman'scostume.

White shamans get their magical power from a westerly direction, the home of the benevolent deities and spirits. They operated at a tribal level almost only as healers and diviners and they only had dealings with beneficent entities. It was their role to pacify angry or evil spirits, exorcise them if they possessed human beings and help the tribe live in harmony with their natural environment and the spirit world. On a physical level, they were often employed in an administrative role to oversee tribal affairs.[150]

To the Black Shamans, who epitomized courage and iron discipline, the White Shamans personified humanity. Instead of pitting force against force and bad against bad, like the Black Shamans, the White Shamans had a set of beliefs and customs related to White deeds, habits, and thoughts. In ancient times, the White Shamans created rituals that called upon the peaceful masters or spirits of the White Side; only directing their worship and prayers in this direction. Mongolian shamans became divided into black and white factions. [151]

According to the surviving sources, White Shamans were relatively many. They carried out activities and rituals concerning the general direction peoples' lives were taking most directly through keeping public and administrative order. They instructed people to commune with nature, water, and earth spirits; pacifying angry spirits and undoing the damage they caused. White Shamans also cared for the health of the people. [152]

White Shamans do not use the same tools as Black shaman, for example, they do not use a drum. Instead, they walk with a wooden staff and ring bells during ceremonies. There are also differences in the costume worn by White Shamans. They do not wear antlered headdress, instead they wear a cape called a nemerge.

Buddhist Lamaism was the major cause of the decline in the numbers of White shamans. During the 17th to 19th centuries, the White shaman tradition suffered most among the Khalka and Barga tribes, and throughout Inner Mongolia. In the present day, white shamanism is returning.

---

[150] https://www.newdawnmagazine.com/articles/secrets-of-siberian-shamanism, SecretsofSiberianShamanism.
[151] https://mongolianstore.com/the-black-shamans/, TheBlackandWhiteShamans.
[152] https://mongolianstore.com/the-black-shamans/, TheBlackandWhiteShamans.

Yellow shamanism is the term used to designate a particular version of shamanism practised in Mongolia and Siberia which incorporates rituals and traditions from Buddhism. "Yellow" shows Buddhism in Mongolia, since most Buddhists there belong to what is called the "Yellow sect" of Tibetan Buddhism, whose members wear yellow hats during services. The term also serves to distinguish it from shamanism not influenced by Buddhism (according to its adherents), called "Black Shamanism."[153]

The term "yellow shamanism" was first introduced in 1992 by Sendenjav Dulam and its use then adopted by Otgony Pürev, who considers it to b4e the Buddhism-influenced successor of an unbroken practice that goes back to Genghis Khan—that earlier practice was "black shamanism" and was practised by the Darkhad in defiance of the Buddhism introduced to the area by the Khalka. According to Pürev, the centre of yellow shamanism was the Dayan Deerh monastery in Khövsgöl Province, where he found evidence of yellow practices in the recitations and prayers of a shaman born in the province in 1926; he argues that yellow shamanism has by now ceased to exist anywhere.

Between the 17th and 19th centuries, Lamaism, Tibetan Buddhism[154] imposed itself on the people of Mongolia. Although not the state religion as it was in Tibet, Buddhist persecution made it very difficult for shamans of all beliefs. Black shamans who refused to submit to the foreign religion. White shamans were divided. Some submitted to Buddhist authority and became Yellow shamans. Other White shamans refused to give up their traditions. These shamans were thrown into the "Black" category by the Lamaists.[155] Therefore, both Black and White shamans were in the same category between the 17th and 19th centuries.

Yellow Shaman are those who are controlled by Buddhist Lamas, and practise shamanic rituals and traditions with Tibetan Buddhism.

After the establishment of the Great Mongol Empire of Chinggis Khan, his Borjigin clan became the Golden (Imperial) clan, towering above all Mongol clans. The Lord-Spirits, the Protector-Spirits, the Guardian-Spirits of the BorJigin clan were raised to the high rank of the Ancestor-Spirits of the whole nation of Mongols.

The establishment of Buddhism in Mongolia and the adoption of Buddhism by the Borjigin clan resulted in White Shamans and Shamanesses accepting willingly the new Yellow Religion, "Yellow" being the Saffron colour of Buddhist robes. White Shamans and Shamanesses embracing Buddhism received the title "Yellow Shamans and Shamanesses." Black Shamans and Shamanesses did not/do not accept Buddhism.
Many of these Yellow Shamans and Shamanesses had the books of shamanist prayers and hymns in Mongolian transcribed by monks with the Tibetan syllabic characters as Buddhist books of prayers, and the monks and Yellow Shamans believed that a Mongol text transcribed with Tibetan characters is eight times more blessed than the same text written in Mongol letters. [156]

---

[153] Wikipedia, Yellowshamanism.
[154] Wikipedia, TibetanBuddhism.
[155] Wikipedia, TibetanBuddhism.
[156] Yönsiyebü Rinchen, "White, Black and Yellow Shamans Among the Mongols," *Ultimate Reality and Meaning* 4, no. 2 (1981), https://doi.org/10.3138/uram.4.2.94.

Because of this, the distinctions between the two traditions were Muddied in Lamaist dominated regions. Luckily, the tribes in the northwest regions such as the Darhad and Urinahai had close contact and solidarity with Siberian peoples such as the Tuvans and Buryats, who kept their traditions intact.

Communism in Mongolia stopped the Buddhist atrocities, but was a step backwards for freedom of religion. When Mongolia changed to a democracy in the 1990s, shamanism grew stronger in the region again.

"White shamans," have returned and are no longer forced into the "Yellow" category. The "Yellow"

Table 3 The Buddhist concept of 9 levels of Consciousness.

Consciousness	Physically	Description	
1st Level	Sight	What we See	
2nd Level	Hearing	What we Hear	
3rd Level	Smell	What we Smell	
4th Level	Taste	What we Taste	
5th Level	Touch	What we Touch	
6th Level	The 6th Sense integrates the first five levels of Consciousness into a whole. We make judgements and take action here. This is our consciousness mind		
7th Level	The intuitive realm where we self-identify and distinguish ourselves from others		
8th Level	Our Karmic energy store house. It is here the latent causes and effects of our thoughts, words and deeds accumulate. This level is eternal.		
9th Level	Pure life force, the power to live . . . It is the greater self that works for the happiness of all		

category is no longer a shaman classification.

S hamanism is universal and not bound by social or cultural conditions. It is the most ancient and most enduring spiritual tradition known to humanity. Shamanism predates and makes up the foundation of all known religions or religious philosophies.[157]

In the Shaman's world view, spirits and demons inhabit everything around us. Every part of the natural environment is alive with different sentient forces. Literally, the world is alive, in the mountains, trees, rivers and lakes, rocks, fields, the sky, and the earth. There are supernatural spirits and souls. Added to this, each region has its own native spiritual beings, and people living in those areas are powerfully aware of their presence. In order to stay in the spirit's good graces, offerings are made, rituals performed and sometimes people will refrain from particular places to avoid the more dangerous forces.

The focus of Buddhist teaching and practice is centred on commonplace goals, seeking advice from shamans whose function is to contact spirits, to predict their influences on people's lives, and to perform rituals that either overcome harmful influences or otherwise ask for their help makes sense. Making such request and receiving a shaman's aid should give people a measure of control over their unpredictable lives and surroundings.

Rituals conducted today have changed from those of previous centuries. Not that they are any less effective today. They are. But the style and form of them from previous centuries have changed. Comparing rituals and practices from previous generations or those performed centuries ago to today makes little sense.

When Tonpa Shenrab came to Tibet which, according to the well-known 20th-century Buddhist scholar Gedun Chophel he blessed Tibet and its people, sharing many teachings, ceremonies and religious dances that are distinctly Bon. The most important change he introduced was to eliminate animal sacrifices. The local practice was to sacrifice animals in order to appease spirits responsible for causing sickness and misfortune. Tonpa Shenrab taught them they could offer red torma and white torma in place of animals. Torma is figures made mostly of flour and butter used in tantric rituals or as offerings in Tibetan Buddhism. They may be dyed in different colours, often with white or red for the main body of the torma. They are made in specific shapes based on their purpose, usually conical in form.[158] In this way, Tonpa Shenrab established the peaceful, enlightened Yungdrung-Bon tradition. [159]

The Shaman is contemporary to the world they live in. They wear clothes and use tools and aids suitable to the society and expectations of their clients. To bring "bear" energy to his or her client, the shaman may wear something to connect with that animal or spirits energy. A bear claw beneath the shirt or wrap a subtle piece of fur around their rattle handle would be acceptable.

The shaman believes they are talking to guides, perhaps spirits, and those spirits can help them heal. In order to heal, the shaman must be able to connect with the recipient of the healing. This means the recipient of healing needs to be open to receiving it.

---

[157] shamanicdrumming.com, ShamanicDrumming.
[158] Wikipedia, Torma.
[159] buddhaweekly.com/, linterview-bon-teacher-chaphur-rinpoche-explains-bon-different-similar-five-buddhist-schools-tibet.

If a shaman hasn't aligned with practices and rituals of a particular culture, preferring to belong to the one of their birth, they are considered being contemporary shaman and needs to be authentic and able to communicate this to the recipient and for the information to be accepted.

Direct connection with the spirits is through song and dance. The rhythm of the music, song and dance take the shaman into a state of ecstasy where he, or she, is in direct communion with the spirits, they go beyond ordinary human existence and reach a transcendental state of simultaneous existence in this world and the next, and bring him back with messages and information. They also close the session with the spirits and his souls returns to him.

24.1 Drums and Drumstick

Usually, the shaman's drum is a fixture of their healing ceremonies and has special qualities. It has been blessed by the shaman who owns and uses it only. A spirit may exist in the drum that helps the shaman in releasing part of his soul into the journeys he undertakes when it is used. Drumming has a specific role to play in a ceremony.

A slow repetitive drumming rhythm with a frequency close to that measured from the earth has proved effective for most people. It helps induce a range of ecstatic trance states in order to connect with the spiritual dimension of reality. Practised in diverse cultures around the planet, this drum method is strikingly similar to the world over.

Just the way a soothing song can help someone achieve a calmer state. The rhythm of the drum puts you in the right state to journey. The drum beat used is very close to the frequency that is measured from the earth, and has proved effective for most people.

As the Shaman transits through different trance states, the drumming rhythm changes. Eventually, the shaman reaches the level necessary for healing to take place. The drumming tempo will change and slow down when the shaman preparing to leave the trance state. The change in tempo helps draw their consciousness back to normal.

Power animal drumming is a shamanic way to evoke and internalize animal archetypes. An animal archetype represents the spirit and attributes of the entire species of that animal. Shamanism is the endeavour to cultivate ongoing relationships with power animals to gain insight, healing methods, and other vital information that can benefit the community. When an animal spirit is invoked, there is often an accompanying rhythm that comes through. Shamans frequently use these unique rhythms to summon their helping spirits for the work at hand. 160

24.2 Songs

The most important thing about a shamanic song is whether it is effective.

The purpose of the shamanic song is to connect to, and bring in different energies. The purpose of the singing that song is to shift one's state of mind and the state of the group that is singing. The song doesn't have to be beautiful, or perfectly written. The power of the song is the doorway that it opens between the shaman or the individuals and the power of the spirit world. That doorway is actually open by the singer(s), not the song itself. Some songs are more effective at helping you open that door.[161]

Shamanic songs can be unique to individual healers and/or groups of people. They really aren't different from any spiritual song. Often, the shaman will go to the spirit world to get the lyrics or melody of the song. They may have an occasion or a purpose and they will consult with the spirit world to be inspired by a song that fits well with what they want to do.

In terms of spiritual practice, there are many healthful benefits to singing, and positive purposes for singing. Here are some of those benefits: [162]

---

[160] shamanicdrumming.com, ShamanicDrumming.
[161] shamanlinks.net, SingingShamanicSongs-ShamanLinks.
[162] shamanlinks.net, SingingShamanicSongs-ShamanLinks.

- Singing is a powerful way of filling yourself with good energy.

- Singing can help you change your emotions or your state of mind.

- Shamans use songs to help groups harmonize their energy with one another.

- Singing can help you connect with a higher power, such as angels, or guardian spirits, or the divine (in whatever way you name it).

- You can use singing to bring good energy into a room. In some spiritual practices, songs are used to invoke or invite. For instance, there are songs for rain, or songs for inviting a power animal to be with you.

- Many shamans have a healing song that they sing when they work with their clients.

- Songs can bless another person or a group of people.

- Singing can connect you to the deeper knowing that is inside of you.

- Songs can help you release or express feelings or stuck energies you have found it difficult to release or express by thinking or talking about them.

- Songs can heal you.

24.3 Dance

Dance is a creative activity. A shaman will add dance to their drumming and singing to bring spirits into our world. These are spirits they have asked their helping spirits to bring for healing. Physically moving the human body requires energy, coordination and strongly reinforces the request and connection. It adds a mutual energy exchange between the shaman and the spirits they are dancing with.

When the spirit is an animal, certain steps and actions during the dance will mimic and imply the spirit of the animal the shaman is connected with.

Dance is also a traditional element of spiritual practice. The intention and form of the dance may have a specific purpose. A dance may start as a method of connecting to and invoking spirits for the healing that is requested. Later, toward the end of the dance, the message to the spirits may be one of thanks for attending and taking part in the ceremony.

Some shaman will dance because they enjoy dancing with their spirits and guides and this personal connection through motion and energy is an important way to express and enjoy their connection.

25   Costumes

All parts of the costume are personal to the shaman. A shaman's costume is not bought off the shelf, it is made on the direction of the spirits and the spirit world the shaman journeys to. It is made of time and may have things added to it and taken away depending on the humanizing the shaman is undertaking.

The other aspect of the costume is the self-training wearing the costume instill on the shaman. By putting on the costume, they are communicating to themselves the role they are taking on, the power they are seeking to accept and connect with and also the start of the session. By taking it off, they are leaving the session and the connection.

25.1   Headband and Headdress

Feathers symbolize flight, travel, and the ability of the shaman to travel with and to the spirits he or she must visit in the upper or lower worlds to discover the cause of what is afflicting the recipient and how healing is to be achieved. Feathers from powerful birds, especially predators such as Eagles instill power into the headdress and the shaman's connection to these animals.

If the shaman's power animal is a bird, feathers or claws of the bird are an essential part of the headdress and show honour and the state of their connectedness because the shaman is wearing aspects of the physical animal.

Other symbolize can be communicated in the headdress. The four seasons, the four directions, certain elements. Parts of the Shamanic cosmos can also appear. Even the DNA spiral can be added to a modern shaman's headdress and headband.

A headband may have cords or tassels hanging down which cover the face and form a screen which prevents people from seeing the shaman's face. There are three reasons usually offered for this:

1. The shaman will take on the characteristics of their helping spirit or guide. This may include the face of a guide that has long since passed over. People seeing this altered face would/might be scared. The screen hides the face of the spirit from onlookers.

2. The cords and tassels symbolize the nature of the two worlds. The physical world is on our side of the cord screen, the shaman, is on the other side, soul journeying in another realm.

3. Distraction. The screen removes the physical world from the shaman's gaze, removing what is taking place around him, allowing him to blend and connect with the spirit world more effectively.

25.2   Cloak

As with the headdress and headband, there are no strict guidelines on how to build and what should be represented on such a shamanic garment. It should include more connections to their power animal and spirits they are connected with. This may mean duplicating some aspects of the headdress and headband, but reinforcement of these helping spirits is very acceptable.

They are allies and helpers in the spirit world, expressing the connection cannot be done too often!

The cloak also represents energy, a shield against harmful or malevolent spirits the shaman may encounter. Some shaman, at the direction of their helping spirts may attach panels of highly polished metal to their cloak. The metal acts as a mirror.

A malevolent spirit seeking to attack the shaman will see themselves in the mirror and become confused and leave. Metal is used, because a piece of an actual mirror may break and become useless. Shards of glass are also dangerous to the shaman if the malevolent spirt uses a piece to attack the shaman. Bells and metal made to rattle can be attached to scare away harmful spirits.

25.3 Foot Wear

During shamanizing, dancing, and soul journeying, strong, protective footwear is required! Footwear, usually some sort of boots can be decorated with symbols and elements of power animals, helping spirits and guides. Something like these boots will bring me home. But also, if during a soul journey the shaman must cross a river, walk on water, or across rough ground, suitable footwear is required.

25.4 Alters and Shrines

Alters and shrines in a home or shamanic place of healing reinforce the shamans power animal, and all helping spirits. Metal mirrors may be on display to ward off and confuse any dark or lower spirits which may seek to harm the shaman as he prays.

Members of the shaman's family may be represented, especially if those family members were shamans, their energy and strength can be called on to help the living shaman. Food offering and offerings of other acceptable gifts to the spirits will be displayed and available for the spirits to consume.

Representation of local spirits associated with the spiritual beings of the area where the shaman is living will be important. When humans build houses or even set down a temporary abode, we disrupt the spirits in the local area. By showing them on the altar, we honour them and ask for their agreement to us staying there.

S hamanic mirrors are metallic discs made of bronze or other metals, polished on one side, their "face" and usually decorated on the "back." In the centre of the back, there is often a knob or boss with a hole through it. This hole is to allow a cord, silk ribbon or scarf to be passed through it, which enables the mirror to be suspended or tied to a costume, hung over a shaman alter, or, if small enough attached to a shaman's costume. The cord, ribbon or scarf allows the mirror to be handled without torching the polished reflective surface.

The face of a bronze mirror is convex, although some are flat. Concave mirrors are rare. Historically, in ancient China household fires were kept alive both day and night throughout the year to cook, heat water and for warmth. However, once a year the fires had to be put out. The next day, at noon, new fires were ceremonially lit by a shaman or priest, who used a concave bronze mirror. When using such a mirror, the sun's rays are reflected into a single point, which generates enough heat to light some kindling. Today we can achieve the same result by the use of a glass lens. Himalayan melong[163] mirrors, with a bronze loop on their top edge, are sometimes polished on both sides. These are convex on the one face, and concave on the other. As a heart protecting mirror, the convex side is worn outward. For divination, the convex side is to see into the future, and the concave side to see into the past.[164]

The origin of ceremonial mirrors developed in Neolithic times with the art of grinding and polishing stone. Obsidian and jade were often used in ancient mirrors, and these stones are found in different locations around the world, such as Mexico, Anatolia and China. Polished, iron-rich meteorites may also predate cast bronze mirrors, and these have been used for a very long time in Tibet to create mirrors and other sacred objects.

Over the millennia shamans found many ways to use their mirrors. Some shaman mirrors are often known as toli[165] and give spirits a house to live in. Some shamans use them by entering a trance and working with the energies amplified by, or inherently present, in the mirror. Shamans use them for performing healings, for exorcism, for soul retrieval.

A toli is a round, ritual mirror used in Shamanism in some parts of Mongolia and in the Republic of Buryatia. The mirror, ornamented on one side with depictions of animals, plants, birds and polished on the other, may be made of bronze, brass or copper.

Small Toli is traditionally worn as part of a shaman's attire around the shaman's neck, or in quantity on the shaman's kaftan or apron which is often referred to as their armour. These pieces of ritual clothing help to protect the shaman from hostile spirit attack. Toli help ward off harmful or attacking spirits in their own right, and can also be thought of as an object which signifies the shaman's authority or role. [166]

One role of the Toli is as heart protector. The toli must be large enough to cover a shaman's heart and the cord, scarf, or ribbon must be long enough for the mirror to rest over the heart, a vital organ and one that evil spirits will attack. Smaller mirrors, just a few centimetres across may be

---

[163] Wikipedia, Melong.
[164] http://www.greenshinto.com/wp/2016/03/12/zen-and-shinto-10-more-mirrors/, ZenandShinto ShamanMirrorsGreenShinto.
[165] Wikipedia, Tolishamanism.
[166] Wikipedia, Tolishamanism.

attached to the shaman's costume or be set into wooden handles which the shaman can hold. The belief is that an evil spirt will see their reflection in the mirror and be terrified and run away.

When a shaman dies, it is traditional for their body, mirrors, drums and other sacred items to be taken to a remote location and set out on a platform in a tree. Later generations of shamans may accidentally "find" the deceased's mirrors and other bronze objects, and after consulting the spirit of the deceased shaman to ask for permission to adopt the mirror, the shaman who found these ancient objects could use them in his own work.

Himalayan melong[167] mirrors, with a bronze loop on their top edge, are sometimes polished on both sides. These are convex on the one face, and concave on the other. [168]

Tibetan Buddhism or Lamaism is a blend of Buddhism that entered Tibet in the 8th century and shamanism. The unique blend found in Tibet, has followers in Mongolia, China and Nepal. In this tradition, mahasiddhas[169] great adepts or mystics, oracles and healers all have melongs or "heart protecting mirrors."

A. Mahasiddha is someone who embodies and cultivates the "siddhi[170] of perfection." A siddha[171] is an individual who, attains the realization of siddhis, psychic abilities and powers. Mahasiddhas were practitioners of yoga and Tantra, or tantrikas. Their historical influence throughout the Indian subcontinent and the Himalayas was vast, and they reached mythic proportions as codified in their songs of realization and hagiographies, or namtars, many of which have been preserved in the Tibetan Buddhist canon. The Mahasiddhas are the founders of Vajrayana[172] traditions and lineages such as Dzogchen[173] and Mahamudra.[174]

The 9th-century Borobudur stupa in Java shows the Buddha surrounded by monks, who are lifting their handled mirrors, to charge them with the high energy of his enlightened being.
This use of mirrors as a sort of "sacred battery" which holds a spiritual charge also occurs in medieval Europe as Christian relics were sometimes viewed in a mirror, the mirror capturing and holding the reflection of the sacred relic for the pilgrim to take away with them.[175]

Large alter mirrors are displayed on Buddhist alters to symbolize radiant emptiness. A shaman will display their alter mirror on their shamanic alter because it is the honoured home of their helping spirits and as a symbol of their shamanic power.

Shamanic ritual mirrors are living things. Not only do they contain helping spirits and a master spirit. The mirror is cleaned, stored and also dressed according to the instructions of the Master Spirit. Listening to the mirror will cause instructions on how to work with it and the spirits to which it is home, this includes any offerings they require. Traditional offerings to mirrors are incensed, juniper

---

[167] Wikipedia, Melong.
[168] http://www.greenshinto.com/wp/2016/03/12/zen-and-shinto-10-more-mirrors/, ZenandShinto ShamanMirrorsGreenShinto.
[169] Wikipedia, Mahasiddha.
[170] Wikipedia, Siddhi.
[171] Wikipedia, Siddha.
[172] The Mirror, 'TheTibetanBookoftheDead'andVajrayana.
[173] Wikipedia, Dzogchen.
[174] Wikipedia, Mahasiddha.
[175] http://www.greenshinto.com/wp/2016/03/12/zen-and-shinto-10-more-mirrors/, ZenandShinto ShamanMirrorsGreenShinto.

or sage smoke, alcohol—vodka—songs and the sounds of drums rattles and bells.[176] In Mongolia, shamans mirrors were, and still are, blooded in the blood of a sacrificed sheep. The blood is said to transfer the life force of the animal to the mirror.

A shamanic mirror is dressed in silk. The colours of the silk represent both the five elements and the sacred directions. Spirits may request additional offerings to be attached to their mirror, such as beads, stones, shells or small bells, too.

Bronze is an alloy of copper and tin; the percentage of tin varies from between 10% and 30%. The tin content changes the colour and hardness of the bronze; for example, a high level of tin makes the mirror brittle, and it will be prone to break easily, whereas a low level of tin gives a warm red shine, but will easily oxidize. A mirror that is brittle is not desirable. If an evil spirit confronts the shaman, it could break or shatter the mirror, leaving the shaman without heart protection. For this reason, glass is also not used as part of a shaman's mirror. A mirror that has oxidized will affect its reflectivity and, therefore, its ability to scare away an evil spirit when it sees its reflection.

Gold, silver, lead and sometimes zinc can be added to the bronze, which all influence the resulting bronze medal. In the Tibetan language, there are five different words for bronze. Incorporating metal donated by the shaman who will use the mirror creates a bond between the mirror and the shaman practitioner.

---

[176] http://www.greenshinto.com/wp/2016/03/12/zen-and-shinto-10-more-mirrors/, ZenandShinto ShamanMirrorsGreenShinto.

As noted in the sections on Witch Doctors and Medicine People, they are not shaman, calling any other indigenous traditional healer a shaman is also not correct. The shamans discussed and their heritage is in Tibet, Nepal, and on the Mongolian Plain and Siberia.

In those regions, the shamans have filled many roles in history. In their societies, they have been a traditional healer, spiritual leader, ritualist, soul guide, sacrificer, song reciter, dancer, and dramatic performer, confident and even a tribal leader.

In a trance, they would journey to other realms, sometimes dangerous realms. On those journeys, they were guided by spirits and animals; they retrieved souls that had become lost or even stolen. They journey to find and discover the cause of illness and how to remedy and heal the recipient.

These abilities, ceremonies and paraphernalia have made shaman targets for persecution and mistreatment as "modern" western religions connected with shamans. Drums, ceremonial clothing, and all evidence of the shaman's ability were burned and destroyed. Baptism was enforced.

Perhaps worse, denigration of shamans as lesser people, themselves by calling them by disrespectful names and labels such as devils, demons, and assigning them a lower rank or status in society.

The twentieth century misapplication of the word shaman to other cultural heritages denigrates the word and the societies to which it rightfully applies as well as those it does not.

Persecution of Siberian shamans and prohibition of shamanic ceremonies began in 17th century Siberia at the time orthodox Christianity was forced on the population. Yet, it failed to eradicate shamanism. Many Russians, even czarist officials, turned to shamanic practitioners for the advice and help and availed themselves of the shaman's otherworldly capabilities.

Declining religious influence, especially Judo-Christian churches in the Western world, has coincided with the realignment of shamanism by scientific investigation and reporting who now see the shaman as a neuropsychiatric healer.

During a shamanic ceremony, the shaman will enter an altered state of consciousness ASC. The ASC is often referred to as an ecstatic state. It is during this time that they connect with the other realms they are journeying to, their helping spirits and the gods and spirits that will help them, help the recipient, on whose behalf they are making this journey.

The ecstatic state also describes a dislocation between the physical individual that is the shaman in the ceremony and the soul of a person journeying to another realm. The ASC, or trance state, allows the shaman to journey from their physical existence to the destination they need to go. This may involve flying, that is transforming themselves into a bird or riding on an animal. In this journey, there is no restriction on which of the worlds they can go to; upper, middle for lower. They simply go where they are needed or choose to go.

Lower world journeys are usually in cases of soul retrieval, see later, or to bring a dead person's soul to Erleg Khan.

A common metaphor for a journey such as this is an Out of Body experience commonly reported by many people. In an out-of-body experience, there are two souls or beings exist, the physical one and the ephemeral one that can journey across the room, look at a room from a different perspective or across the world. Military forces, notably the US and Russians, have experimented with "remote viewing" of each other's secret sites and have done so for decades.

In shamanic ceremonies, the ASC state is self-induced by the shaman and the western medical background has frequently attributed psychopathology to actions and expressions of shamanic practitioners in such an ASC; of shaman candidates during their initiatory period and of performing shamans during their ceremonies.

During an ASC trance, a shaman may utter animal sounds as transformations in order to original spirits occur. He/She may appear unconscious in this world as certain stages of the journey take place. If the shaman is dancing or drumming, the speed and rhythm may change according to the progress made.

Most Altaic[177] shamans speak of passing nine landmarks during their journey regardless of which world they travel in.

Most traditional non-Western cultures and in historical European cultures, ASC are or were interpreted either as a special state of the individual permitting of close interaction with supernatural entities, in order to receive their messages, perceive them in visions, and gain power from them; or, as a state of possession in which a supernatural entity or power acts through the individual.[178]

It is worth noting at this point that the shaman is not possessed. Shamanism is not a possession state belief. Shamanic possession is not actually possession at all, but the intentional embodiment of spirit helps with whom the shaman has already developed a working relationship. Possession is the unintentional intrusion of a foreign spirit into a person who is considered an energetic illness or unhealthy state in shamanism. Embodiment is an effective, working, altered state. The shaman can begin and end at will.
Shamanism and possession share biological features in their elicitation of ancient brain systems to change the consciousness in relation to healing and spiritual experiences.

Shamans are chosen by a spirit, or the show the ability to connect with the other realms and spirits but have no reference to do so and no way of organizing and managing what is happening to them. This is not a role people can vie for like a class president. There is no written exam mark to be passed. The initiatory sickness as it is called takes many forms depending on the person being called and their circumstances. Nervous fits, attacks of insanity, loss of consciousness, epileptic convulsions and experiences of being torn apart or dismembered are some of them. In the 2000s the experience and reference points will differ from those of hundreds of years ago. Recovery from the sickness is presented by shaman teachers as death and rebirth; being reborn to the shamanic vocation as a changed person.[179]

---

[177] Wikipedia, Altaiclanguages.
[178] WOLFGANG G. JILEK, TransformingtheShamanChangingWesternViewsofShamanismandAlteredStatesofConsciousness.
[179] JILEK, TransformingtheShamanChangingWesternViewsofShamanismandAlteredStatesofConsciousness.

On the individual and interpersonal level, shamanic practitioners, unlike Western-trained health professionals, combine the confidence-inspiring reputation of a charismatic personality with access to supernatural powers and a culture-congenial understanding of their clients' belief and value system. [180]

All this may explain the survival of shamanic practices among indigenous peoples despite centuries of suppression by governmental and ecclesiastical authorities. However, beyond mere survival, we witness a revival of shamanic healing rituals and ceremonialism, especially among North American indigenous populations under Westernizing acculturation pressure. This indigenous renaissance is reflected in the revitalization of traditional ceremonials with important therapeutic aspects throughout North America.

Examples are the Winter Spirit Dances of the Salish in the Pacific Northwest; the Sun Dance among aboriginal populations of Wyoming, Idaho, Utah, Colorado, and the Dakotas; the Gourd Dance among the Kiowa, Comanche, Cheyenne, and Arapaho, which subsequently reached many other tribes in the United States and Canada; the Peyote Cult, which spread northward from Mexico and is today a major pan-Amerindian religious ceremonial east of the Rocky Mountains. [181]

In North America, the expansion of rituals and ceremonies speaks to the need for indigenous people to have an identity unique to themselves. Preserving and expanding the role of traditional healers is a powerful way of expressing this voice while allowing for modern medicine to intervene where necessary.

In reading and exploring the role of Tibetan Shaman, and Shamanism at the roof of the world. Shaman there do not diagnose and will send a potential client to a doctor to get antibiotics or more expensive treatment.

Beginning in the later part of the 1900s what we call "New Age" shamanism has appeared and taken hold in people and places without the indigenous or traditional heritage associated with shamanism.

This profound and honest interest in shamanism in cultures that do not have a historical connection to shamanism is because of an enquiring mind and desire to understand and the feeling that there is more to what I know and understand. Shamanism would not have survived from the Paleolithic without it having substance to it.

The revival of shamanic ceremonialism is one aspect of the renaissance of indigenous culture. This occurred in the aftermath of decolonization, accompanied by a profound change in the prevailing Western attitudes after World War II. There has been a change in the world view and a sense of superiority. No longer are Europe or North America the centre for everything that is right and correct, and prepared to remake everything in their image. Today they are the source of financial resources, powerful inquisitiveness, and a desire to explore and understand.

---

[180] JILEK, TransformingtheShamanChangingWesternViewsofShamanismandAlteredStatesofConsciousness.
[181] JILEK, TransformingtheShamanChangingWesternViewsofShamanismandAlteredStatesofConsciousness.

28 Persecution of Shaman

28.1 Religious Persecution in Tibet

Current religious persecution in Tibet does not stem from ethnic or religious conflict or discrimination by a majority against a minority. It is politically motivated, and consciously applied to realize political and military ends.

28.2 History

The Tibetan Plateau has been inhabited by humans for at least 21,000 years. The Neolithic period saw immigrants from northern China largely displace the humans around 3,000 years ago. There remains some genetic continuity between the Paleolithic inhabitants and contemporary Tibetan populations.[182]

The earliest Tibetan historical texts identify the Zhang Zhung culture as a people who migrated from the Amdo region into what is now the region of Guge in western Tibet. Zhang Zhung is considered to be the original home of the Bon religion.

By the 1st century BCE—Before Common Era[183], a neighbouring kingdom arose in the Yarlung Valley, and the Yarlung king, Drigum Tsenpo, attempted to remove the influence of the Zhang Zhung by expelling the Zhang Bon priests from Yarlung. He was assassinated and Zhang Zhung continued its dominance of the region until it was annexed by Songtsen Gampo in the 7th century. Prior to Songtsen Gampo, the kings of Tibet were more mythological than factual, and there is insufficient evidence of their existence.

The fall of the Tibetan Empire[184] resulted in the region breaking up into a variety of territories each controlled by a warlord with overall influence being either Mongol or Chinese but with a reasonable amount of self-determination and flexibility. Eventually, with the fall of the Mongol empire and influence, Tibet was absorbed into the Chinese provinces of Sichuan and Qinghai. Generally, the current borders of Tibet were determined by the 18th century.

In 1950, The Peoples Republic of China negotiated an agreement with the newly enthroned 14th Dalai Lama affirming China's sovereignty over Tibet. Autonomy Created the Tibet Autonomous Regional [TAR] and the head of the government to be ethnic Tibetan. In reality the actual power in the TAR is the First Secretary of the Tibet Autonomous Regional Committee of the Chinese Communist Party, who has never been a Tibetan. The role of ethnic Tibetans in the higher levels of the TAR Communist Party remains very limited.
In exile, the Dalai Lama[185] repudiated the agreement. Many Tibetans have fled Tibet to Nepal and India. The Dalai Lama has a strong following, many Tibetan look at him as both a political and a spiritual leader.

A rival Tibetan government-in-exile, The Central Tibetan Administration, also referred to as The Tibetan Government in Exile is located in India. Its internal structure is government-like; it has

---

[182] Wikipedia, Tibet.
[183] Wikipedia, CommonEra.
[184] Wikipedia, TibetanEmpire.
[185]

stated that it is "not designed to take power in Tibet"; rather, it will be dissolved as soon as freedom is restored in Tibet in favour of a government formed by Tibetans inside Tibet. In addition to political advocacy, it administers a network of schools and other cultural activities for Tibetans in India. [186]

During the Chinese Cultural Revolution[187] 1959–1961, most of Tibet's more than 6,000 monasteries were destroyed and others severely damaged and defaced by the Communist Party of China and monastic estates were broken up and secular education introduced.[188] During this period, religious objects, of any sort were confiscated and destroyed, removing a significant amount of personally owned history and connection with the past heritage of Tibet.

Restrictions were lifted during the 1980s as a result of a period of relative accommodation but it resulted in a resurgence of religious activity both formal and public as well as personal; Tibetans created altars in their homes, prayed in public, and made pilgrimages to holy places. Rebuilding of temples and monasteries—almost entirely supported by people's voluntary labour and resources. Those monasteries and nunneries were filled with young monks and nuns who wished to pursue a religious vocation in spite of growing up under Communist Chinese rule.

In 1987 and subsequent years, arrest of monks, nuns, and the display of images of the Dali Lama, shouting slogans and putting up posters have been instituted. Subsequent economic and other reforms have sought to suppress religious activity and any visible reference to the Dali Lama as a spiritual or political head of Tibet.

28.3 Shamans

Shamanism is the oldest religious activity in humanity, it was and has been effected in two ways.

First, in a community a Shaman is a highly respected and honoured confident, healer, and leader. In both Soviet Russia and China, those roles can be manipulated into a portrayal of the shaman as an oppressor of this tribe or community. They were seen to fall into the same classification as land owners, merchants, local leaders, or aristocracy. In both Soviet Russia and China, Shamans were purged, arrested, tortured and shot along with the other classes of people communist forces saw as being oppressors and inhibiting progress of socialist ideas and disrupting the agricultural and societal changes they wanted to make in the name of state ownership.

Suppression by the Red Army and the People's Liberation Army [China] included not just the shaman, but possessions, all things that formed the shaman's heritage, places of worship. And performance of rituals. Some interesting workarounds to survive the persecution has been recorded. One Shaman in Siberia turned his rituals into what he called a "theatre production" in this way he was providing entertainment rather than say a soul retrieval ritual, if anyone from the local Soviet happened to be in the "audience" and wanted to know. Other Shaman survived by simply being in very remote locations that the communist re-educators and military did not care to go.

[186] Wikipedia, CentralTibetanAdministration.
[187] Wikipedia, CulturalRevolution.
[188] Wikipedia, CulturalRevolution.

In both Soviet Russia and Tibet, the systematic state sponsored destruction of monasteries and arrest of monks and nuns was material to depriving their respective societies of the physical presence of shamans, Bonpo, and Buddhist monks as well as the physical presence of buildings and places of worship.

The heritage and substance of shamanism that had been part of a chain of religious growth, through Bon and ultimately into Tibetan Buddhism with its scholarly monastic environment where practices and beliefs were recorded in books and scripture, was unlike any persecution that had come and gone previously.

The introduction of Russian and Chinese languages with state education to replace shamanic teachings and monastic education has resulted in more than one generation growing up without any connection to traditional shamanic teaching, training and practices, or monastic Buddhist teachings. However, as noted previously this did not prevent people of all ages attempting reconnection with their spiritual and religious heritage.

Since the collapse of the Soviet system in 1991, there has been a resurgence of Shamanic activity in The Mongolian People's Republic. To the point where Shamans advertise, can be members of the Corporate Union of Mongolian Shamans, appear on television and run for local administrative political positions.

However, the loss of people, Shamans, men and women who provided a physical presence and their oral history along with their costumes, drums, altars, and all their paraphernalia cannot be replaced, just as the heritage in the monasteries destroyed by the Chinese communists cannot be replaced.

There are two key differences between the resurgence of Shamanism in Mongolia and Tibet. First, Mongolia is free to determine its own path, and make its own laws and regulations. Second is the deep and magnetic, reverence for Chinggis Khan, or Genghis Khan[189] and the achievement of the Mongol people during the Mongolian Empire is genuine and a source of pride and self-identity.

28.4 Current Threats

Persecution in Soviet Russia and Communist China was systematic, organized, and state sponsored. Shamanism faces new forms of denigration and persecution.

Changes are needed to Western notions of shamanism, the shamanic healer, and the role of altered states of consciousness (ASC). Before the Age of Enlightenment, the shaman was condemned as demoniac charlatan. From the mid-19th until the mid-20th century, the shaman was generally considered as being afflicted with a psychiatric or epileptic condition; a notion based on the misinterpretation of altered states of consciousness in shamanic rituals as psychopathological. [190]

It is worth noting at this point that the shaman is not possessed. Shamanism is not a possession-based belief. Shamanic possession is not actually possession at all, but the intentional embodiment of spirit help with whom the shaman has already developed a working relationship. Possession is unintentional intrusion of a foreign spirit into a person who is considered an energetic

---

[189] Wikipedia, GenghisKhan.
[190] JILEK, TransformingtheShamanChangingWesternViewsofShamanismandAlteredStatesofConsciousness.

illness or unhealthy state in shamanism. Embodiment is an effective, working, altered state the shaman is able to begin and end at will.

Shamanism and possession nonetheless share biological features in their elicitation of ancient brain systems to modify the consciousness in relation to healing and spiritual experiences.

The word shaman has been misapplied to other indigenous healers. This was covered in detail in the first book of The Practical Shaman series. A Shaman is not a Witch Doctor, nor is the Shaman a Medicine Man/Woman.

Neoshamanism refers to "new" forms of shamanism, or methods of seeking visions or healing. Neoshamanism comprises an eclectic range of beliefs and practices that involve attempts to attain altered states and communicate with a spirit world. Neoshamanic systems may not resemble traditional forms of shamanism. Some have been invented by individual practitioners, though many borrow or gain inspiration from a variety of different indigenous cultures. In particular, indigenous cultures of the Americas have been influential. [191]

Neoshamanism is not a single, cohesive belief system, but a collective term for many philosophies and activities. However, certain generalities may be drawn between adherents. Most believe in spirits and pursue contact with the "spirit world" in altered states of consciousness which they achieve through drumming, dance, or the use of entheogens. Most systems might be described as existing somewhere on the animism/pantheism spectrum. Some neoshamans are not trained by any traditional shaman or member of any American indigenous culture, but rather learn independently from books and experimentation. Many attend New Age workshops and retreats, where they study a wide variety of ideas and techniques, both new and old.[192]

Some members of traditional, indigenous cultures and religions are critical of Neoshamanism, asserting that it represents an illegitimate form of cultural appropriation, or that it is nothing more than a ruse by fraudulent spiritual leaders to disguise or lend legitimacy to fabricate, ignorant, and/or unsafe elements in their ceremonies.

According to York (2001) one difference between neoshamanism and traditional shamanism is the role of fear. Neoshamanism and its New Age relations tend to dismiss the existence of evil, fear, and failure. "In traditional shamanism, the shaman's initiation is an ordeal involving pain, hardship and terror. New Age, by contrast, is a religious perspective that denies the ultimate reality of the negative, and this would devalue the role of fear as well."[193]

Inaccurate representation, misrepresentation and careless referencing, attributing actions and belief systems to what is truly a shaman are a danger to shamans everywhere.

---

[191] Wikipedia, Neoshamanism.
[192] Wikipedia, Neoshamanism.
[193] Wikipedia, Neoshamanism.

Bibliography

Ahmad, Feroz. "The Young Turk Revolution." *Journal of Contemporary History* 3, no. 3 (2016): 19-36. https://doi.org/10.1177/002200946800300302.

buddhaweekly.com/. "Iinterview-Bon-Teacher-Chaphur-Rinpoche-Explains-Bon-Different-Similar-Five-Buddhist-Schools-Tibet."

Dictionary, Merriam-Webster. "Definition of Soul by Merriam-Webster."

Dictionary.com. "Aphrodisiac."

———. "Definition of Body at Dictionary.Com."

———. "Incorporeal."

———. "Spirit Definition of Spirit."

Encyclopedia.com. "Shamans."

English, Longman Dictionary of Contemporary. "Spirit Meaning of Spirit."

GotQuestions.org. "What Is the Difference between the Soul and Spirit of Man?".

http://healerofheartsandminds.com. "Reincarnation, Past Lives, Suffering and the Bible, a Shaman's Views."

http://members.tripod.com/infernal_paradise/Wicca.htm. "Wiccan Year."

http://situgen.blogspot.com/search/label/shaman%27s%20costume. "Shaman's Costume."

http://www.face-music.ch/bi_bid/historyoftengerism.html. "Shamanism Tengerism in Mongolia in English."

http://www.greenshinto.com/wp/2016/03/12/zen-and-shinto-10-more-mirrors/. "Zen and Shinto 10 Shaman Mirrors Green Shinto."

https://en.wikipedia.org/wiki/Buryatia. "Buryatia."

https://en.wikipedia.org/wiki/The_City_of_God. "The City of God."

https://mongolianstore.com/the-black-shamans/. "The Black and White Shamans."

https://norse-mythology.org/gods-and-creatures/the-vanir-gods-and-goddesses/freya/. "Freya - Norse Mythology for Smart People."

https://spiritualgrowthguide.com/tengri-shamanism/. "Tengri Shamanism - the Deities of Tengrism - Spiritual Growth Guide."

https://www.allaboutspirituality.org/paganism.htm. "Paganism."

https://www.encyclopedia.com/environment/encyclopedias-almanacs-transcripts-and-maps/ancestors-ancestor-worship. "Ancestors Ancestor Worship.Com."

https://www.energy-shifter.com/shamanism-and-spiritual-techniques.html. "Shamanism, and Soul Retrieval - Spiritual House Cleansing."

https://www.history.com/topics/religion/wicca. "Wicca."

https://www.newdawnmagazine.com/articles/secrets-of-siberian-shamanism. "Secrets of Siberian Shamanism."

https://www.newworldencyclopedia.org/entry/Tengriism. "Tengriism New World Encyclopedia."

International, Pagan Federation. "What Is Paganism."

Jennings, Peter. *Pagan Paths : A Guide to Wicca, Druidry, Asatru, Shamanism and Other Pagan Practices.* London: Rider, 2002.

JILEK, WOLFGANG G. "Transforming the Shaman Changing Western Views of Shamanism and Altered States of Consciousness."

Merriam-Webster. "Definition of New Age."

Mirror, The. "'The Tibetan Book of the Dead' and Vajrayana."

Philosophy, Stanford Encyclopedia of. "Descartes and the Pineal Gland."

Rinchen, Yönsiyebü. "White, Black and Yellow Shamans among the Mongols." *Ultimate Reality and Meaning* 4, no. 2 (1981): 94-102. https://doi.org/10.3138/uram.4.2.94.

shamanicdrumming.com. "Shamanic Drumming."

shamanlinks.net. "Singing Shamanic Songs - Shaman Links."

Wikipeda. "History of the Location of the Soul."

Wikipeda. "Abrahamic Religions."

―――. "Altaic Languages."

―――. "Ancient Greek Religion."

―――. "Animal."

―――. "Animism."

―――. "Atef."

―――. "Banjhakri and Banjhakrini."

―――. "Cathbad."

―――. "Cellular Respiration."

―――. "Central Tibetan Administration."

―――. "Common Era."

―――. "Crook and Flail."

―――. "Cultural Revolution."

―――. "Cybele."

―――. "Dionysus."

―――. "Doreen Valiente."

―――. "Druid."

―――. "Dzogchen."

―――. "Ein Sof."

―――. "Ensoulment."

―――. "Gaul."

―――. "Genghis Khan."

―――. "Gerald Gardner."

―――. "Hinduism."

―――. "History of Anglo-Saxon England."

―――. "Horned God."

―――. "Human Body."

―――. "Indra."

―――. "Irk Bitig."

―――. "Isis."

―――. "Janus."

―――. "Judeo-Christian."

―――. "Kabbalah."

―――. "Khanate."

―――. "List of Neopagan Movements."

―――. "Mahasiddha."

―――. "Mars."

———. "Melong."

———. "Mongols."

———. "Mustafa Kemal AtatüRk."

———. "Neoshamanism."

———. "New Age."

———. "Osiris."

———. "Paganism."

———. "Polytheism."

———. "Ra."

———. "The Secret History of the Mongols."

———. "Seidr."

———. "Seth."

———. "Siddha."

———. "Siddhi."

———. "Soul."

———. "Spirit."

———. "Tengrism."

———. "Tibet."

———. "Tibetan Buddhism."

———. "Tibetan Empire."

———. "Tngri."

———. "Toli Shamanism."

———. "Torma."

———. "Turkic Languages."

———. "Veneration of the Dead."

———. "Viking Age."

———. "Vikings."

———. "Wicca."

———. "Wicker Man."

———. "Xiongnu."

———. "Yellow Shamanism."

www.ingramcontent.com/pod-product-compliance
Lightning Source LLC
Chambersburg PA
CBHW060809270326
41928CB00002B/37